Vascular Access in the Cancer Patient

Alice B. Lucas, R.N., M.B.A.
Vascular Access Nurse Consultant
New York, New York

Elizabeth P. Steinhaus, M.D.
Surgery Branch
National Cancer Institute
Bethesda, Maryland

Michael H. Torosian, M.D.
Associate Professor of Surgery
Division of Surgical Oncology, General Surgery
Hospital of the University of Pennsylvania
Philadelphia, Pennsylvania

Assistant Editor: Eileen Wolfberg
Production Editor: Virginia Barishek
Indexer: Virginia Hobbs
Interior Designer: Chernow Editorial Services, Inc.
Cover Designer: Thomas M. Jackson
Production: Chernow Editorial Services, Inc.
Compositor: The Composing Room of Michigan, Inc.
Printer/Binder: Arcata Graphics/Kingsport

Copyright © 1994, by J. B. Lippincott Company. All rights reserved. No part of this book may be used or reproduced in any manner whatsoever without written permission except for brief quotations embodied in critical articles and reviews. Printed in the United States of America. For information write J. B. Lippincott Company, 227 East Washington Square, Philadelphia, Pennsylvania 19106.

6 5 4 3 2 1

Library of Congress Cataloging-in-Publication Data

Vascular access in the cancer patient : devices, insertion techniques, maintenance, and prevention and management of complications / edited by H. Richard Alexander ; Alice B. Lucas, Elizabeth P. Steinhaus, Michael H. Torosian [contributors].
    p. cm.
  Includes bibliographical references and index.
  ISBN 0-397-51316-X
  1. Cancer—Chemotherapy. 2. Intravenous catheterization.
I. Alexander, H. Richard. II. Lucas, Alice B. III. Steinhaus, Elizabeth P. IV. Torosian, Michael H.
  [DNLM: 1. Catheterization, Central Venous. 2. Catheters, Indwelling—adverse effects. 3. Catheterization, Peripheral. WB 365 V331 1994]
RC271.C5V37 1994
616.99'4061—dc20
DNLM/DLC
for Library of Congress   94-11270
                                                                                 CIP

The authors and publisher have exerted every effort to ensure that drug selection and dosage set forth in this text are in accord with current recommendations and practice at the time of publication. However, in view of ongoing research, changes in government regulations, and the constant flow of information relating to drug therapy and drug reactions, the reader is urged to check the package insert for each drug for any change in indications and dosage and for added warnings and precautions. This is particularly important when the recommended agent is a new or infrequently employed drug.

Vascular Access in the Cancer Patient

Devices, Insertion Techniques, Maintenance, and Prevention and Management of Complications

Edited by

H. Richard Alexander, M.D.
Clinical Assistant Professor of Surgery
Uniformed Services University of the Health Sciences
Senior Investigator
Surgery Branch
National Cancer Institute
Bethesda, Maryland

Four contributors

J.B. Lippincott Company

Philadelphia

*To the clinical associates and nurses of the
National Cancer Institute:*

*"To intervene, even briefly, between our fellow creatures and
their suffering or death, is the most authentic answer to the
question of our humanity."*

Howard Sackler

Preface

It has been estimated that in the United States approximately 500,000 long-term venous access catheters are inserted each year. The widespread use of these catheters since their introduction into clinical practice less than 20 years ago has had an enormous impact on the complexion of cancer treatment. For patients afflicted with cancer, the availability of these devices has provided immeasurable improvement in the quality of life as they provide reliable long-term access to the central venous system and obviate the need for repeated and progressively more difficult venous catheterization and venipuncture. For oncologists, long-term venous access catheters have provided an opportunity to develop increasingly sophisticated, complex, and potentially more effective, treatment protocols. Long-term venous access devices allow oncologic nurses to focus on other important aspects of patient care and monitoring, rather than spend inordinate efforts on simply obtaining and maintaining temporary venous access.

It is incumbent for all health professionals, and for surgeons in particular, because they must expend substantial resources on the insertion and removal of long-term venous access devices and the treatment of device-related complications, to maintain expertise on a variety of topics related to long-term venous access. This includes familiarity with the various features and performance expectations of the different types of catheters available, factors important in appropriate catheter selection, efficient and safe insertion techniques, and routine care and maintenance guidelines. In addition, understanding the principles of diagnosis, treatment, and prophylaxis against complications arising from the use of long-term venous access catheters is important not only to minimize patient morbidity and extend the lifespan of these devices, but also to maximize the efficiency of the resources expended on long-term venous access.

It is for these purposes that this book was written. In this book, one will find a detailed overview of currently available vascular access devices and a review of the comparative features of external catheters versus implantable ports. Standardized approaches to the percutaneous and cutdown insertion techniques as well as alternate insertion options for patients with difficult vascular access are provided in detail. The etiology, diagnosis, treatment, and prophylaxis of catheter-related infectious, occlusive, and thrombotic complications are reviewed in depth but in a format that allows for quick reference to treatment guidelines for any one complication. Finally, information that addresses the rationale behind the routine maintenance of vascular access devices is presented along with guidelines intended to maximize the lifespan of the catheter.

H. Richard Alexander, M.D.

Acknowledgments

The original suggestion for a comprehensive book that addressed all of the aspects involved in the use and care of vascular access devices was made by Dr. Steven A. Rosenberg. It was presented to me by Mr. Stuart Freeman, who is editor of the Oncology Book Division at J. B. Lippincott Company. I am also deeply indebted to Dr. Rosenberg and Dr. Murray Brennan for the initial opportunity and continued privilege of working in the Surgery Branch of the National Cancer Institute. It is very gratifying to see this book published. That it has far exceeded my original expectations is due, in great part, to the fine efforts of my contributors Ms. Alice Lucas, Dr. Betsy Steinhaus, and Dr. Michael Torosian.

At the outset, I woefully underestimated the time required to finish the project. I would be remiss if I did not acknowledge the support and understanding of my lovely wife, Janette. Also, this project would never have been possible without a work environment—in the laboratory and clinics—that was and continues to be extremely stimulating and rewarding. To that end, I thank the very dedicated surgery residents working as research fellows in my laboratory, as well as my colleague and close friend, Dr. Douglas Fraker.

Finally, now that I know what such a project involves, it is clear that I was fortunate to have been associated with J. B. Lippincott Company. Mr. Stuart Freeman provided extremely valuable guidance and just the right nudge at the right time to help me finish the book. Ms. Eileen Wolfberg has been extremely attentive and has often made me feel that this project was her most important assignment. Lastly, I am grateful to Ms. Barbara Owen for her help in typing and preparing the manuscript and Ms. Virginia Barishek for her meticulous and expeditious production of this book.

Contents

1 Long-Term Venous Access Catheters and Implantable Ports 1
   H. Richard Alexander
   Alice B. Lucas

2 Clinical Performance of Long-Term Venous Access Devices 17
   H. Richard Alexander

3 Insertion Technique for Long-Term Venous Access Catheters: Percutaneous Subclavian Vein Cannulation 37
   H. Richard Alexander

4 Long-Term Vascular Access Via Internal Jugular Vein Cutdown 57
   Elizabeth P. Steinhaus

5 Difficult Vascular Access: Alternate Sites and Techniques of Insertion 67
   Michael H. Torosian

6 Thrombotic and Occlusive Complications of Long-Term Venous Access: Diagnosis, Management, and Prophylaxis 89
   H. Richard Alexander

7 Infectious Complications Associated with Long-Term Venous Access Devices: Etiology, Diagnosis, Treatment, and Prophylaxis 111

H. Richard Alexander

8 New Technologies in Long-Term Venous Access and Peripherally Inserted Central Venous Access Catheters 129

H. Richard Alexander
Alice B. Lucas

9 Routine Maintenance and Care of Long-Term Vascular Access Devices 147

Alice B. Lucas

Appendices

A Considerations in Selecting the Appropriate Vascular Access Device 167

B Considerations for Selecting the Most Suitable Site for Long-Term Venous Access 168

C Paradigm for the Evaluation and Treatment of Persistent Withdrawal Occlusion 169

D Paradigm for the Evaluation and Treatment of Partial Catheter Occlusion 170

E Paradigm for the Evaluation and Treatment of Complete Catheter Occlusion 171

F Types and Initial Management of Catheter-Related Infections 172

Index 173

1
Long-Term Venous Access Catheters and Implantable Ports

H. Richard Alexander
Alice B. Lucas

Hickman, Broviac, and Groshong Catheters
Implantable Ports
Other Types of Central Venous Catheters (CVCs)
Repair Kits
References

During the past two decades numerous refinements of existing catheters have been developed and new devices designed to improve clinical performance, reduce complications, and improve patient acceptance of long-term venous access catheters. Broviac introduced the silicone rubber right atrial catheter almost 20 years ago as a less thrombogenic alternative to polyvinyl chloride venous catheters for long-term venous access.[1] Subsequently, the Hickman catheter was introduced as a modification of the Broviac type with a larger internal diameter.[2]

As Hickman catheters initially gained acceptance as an alternative method of venous access in cancer patients, a prospective randomized study was conducted comparing the safety and complications associated with using a Hickman catheter vs multiple temporary polyvinyl chloride central venous catheters in adult cancer patients.[3] Patients requiring long-term venous access (4 to 6 months) were randomly assigned to receive either a Hickman catheter or temporary central venous catheters (CVCs). Thirty Hickman catheters placed in 30 patients had a mean longevity of 188 days and 52 CVCs placed in 18 patients had a mean longevity of 28 days. Technical complications such as cuff extrusion, line fracture, withdrawal occlusion, or catheter occlusion were generally equal between groups. Interestingly, in a situation in which an additional 31 Hickman catheters were placed off-study during the same time period and for which there was significant variability in the method of placement, amount of patient education, and maintenance schedule, there was a higher rate of infectious complications compared to that associated with Hickman catheters placed on-study and for which there was a well-defined maintenance program (Table 1-1). Therefore, when Hickman catheters were utilized within a program of patient education and comprehensive catheter maintenance there appeared to be a low rate of local or systemic infection that was comparable to that observed for CVCs.

Neiderhuber subsequently reported the first series of implantable subcutaneous ports as another method of achieving long-term venous access.[4] In the initial six patients in whom the implantable port was used for venous access, the catheter lumen was small, 0.38 mm, and occlusions developed in five of the six catheters. However, in 19 subsequent patients in whom the port catheter lumen was larger, 0.63 mm, the devices functioned well for an average of 274 ± 110 days. This study established the feasibility of using implantable ports as an alternative method of long-term vascular access.

There appear to be virtually continuous modifications of existing venous access devices with features designed to improve catheter safety and performance. Currently there are basically two types of vascular access devices used for long-term venous cannulation: the external devices such as the Broviac, Hickman, Leonard, or Groshong catheters and the totally implantable venous access ports. The reader is encouraged to review the most recent information on venous access devices at regular intervals to adopt the safest device for use.

TABLE 1-1
Infectious Complication Rate for Hickman Catheters (HC) vs Temporary CVCs: Results of a Prospective Randomized Study

	HC On-study	HC Off-study	CVC On-study
Number of catheters	30	31	52
Superficial infection, n (%)	2 (7)	1 (3)	0 (0)
Catheter sepsis, n (%)	0 (0)	8 (25)*	1 (2)

*Significantly increased incidence of HC-related sepsis in the off-study group by the Fisher exact test. $P<.005$.
Reproduced from Wagman LD, Kirkemo A, Johnston MR. Venous access: a prospective, randomized study of the Hickman catheter. Surgery 1984;95:303–308. Used with permission.

Hickman, Broviac, and Groshong Catheters

The single-lumen Hickman/Broviac type catheter is a barium-impregnated silicone rubber (silastic) catheter and is available as a 2.7-, 4.2-, 6.6-, or 9.6-French device (Figure 1-1). The smaller devices are used primarily for patients in the pediatric age group. The 6.6 and 9.6 Fr catheters are the most widely used single-lumen external type venous access device. The catheters are 90 cm long and can be inserted via

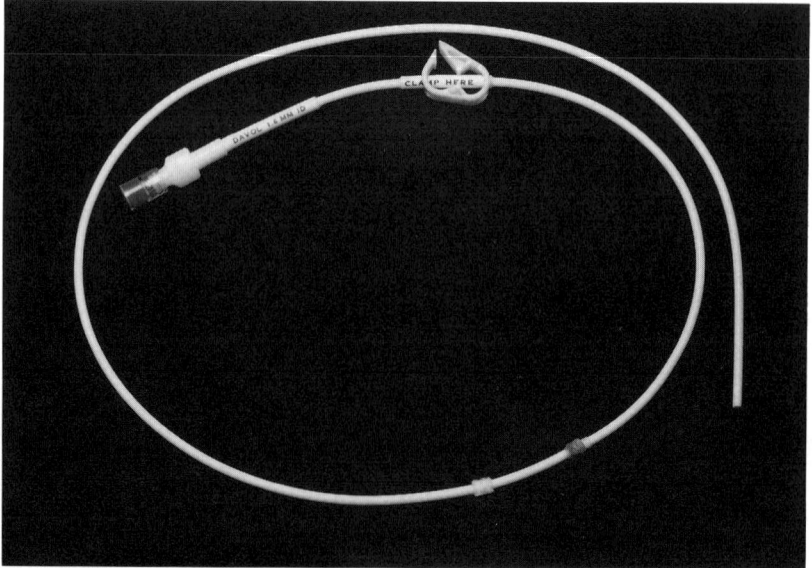

FIGURE 1-1. Single-lumen 9.6-Fr venous access catheter with a 1.6 mm internal diameter. Note the light-colored Dacron cuff and dark-colored silver-impregnated cuff located approximately 30 cm from the external capped hub. Internal length of the catheter is estimated for each patient and cut to appropriate size.

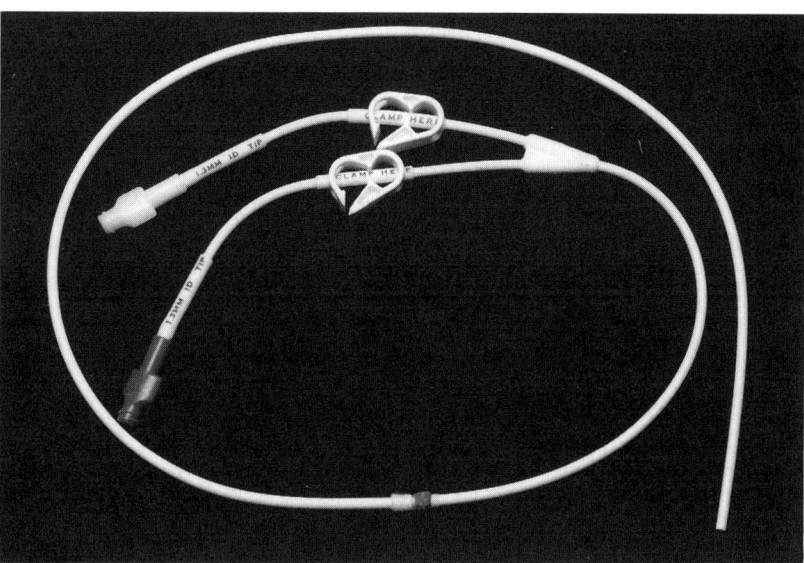

FIGURE 1-2. Double-lumen 10-Fr venous access catheter with Dacron and silver-impregnated cuffs located approximately 30 cm from the external hubs. Note the color coded external hubs are of equal, 1.3 mm internal diameter. Catheter is 90 cm in length and is cut to approximate the appropriate final position in the proximal superior vena caval/right atrial junction. Note reinforced segments for external occluding clamps to prevent catheter fracture.

any venous site (other than distal extremity) and cut to the estimated appropriate length. A Dacron cuff is attached approximately 30 cm from the external hub and is implanted in the subcutaneous tissue just above the exit site. The cuff promotes fibrous ingrowth and scarring which lessens the likelihood of inadvertent catheter removal and prevents bacterial migration along the catheter tunnel. The fibrous ingrowth usually takes from 2 to 6 weeks depending on the patient's condition and not surprisingly the most frequent time for inadvertent catheter removal is within the first 2 weeks of catheter insertion. Also available are catheters with a VitaCuff, a silver-impregnated biodegradable collagen cuff adjacent to the Dacron cuff designed to provide antimicrobial activity for the first 4 to 6 weeks after catheter insertion.

The double-lumen Hickman catheter is available as a 7-, 9-, 10- (Leonard), and 12-Fr catheter. The external adapters on the double-lumen catheter are color coded and of slightly different length so that each channel can be distinguished and they are capped when not in use (Figure 1-2). They are also 90 cm in length and are cut to approximate the appropriate length. The majority of catheters have a double-D configuration (Figure 1-3). The 7- and 9-Fr double-lumen catheters have slightly different internal diameters whereas those of the 10- and 12-Fr catheters are identical. The 10-Fr Leonard catheter has a slightly higher durometer (content) of silicone, making the catheter slightly

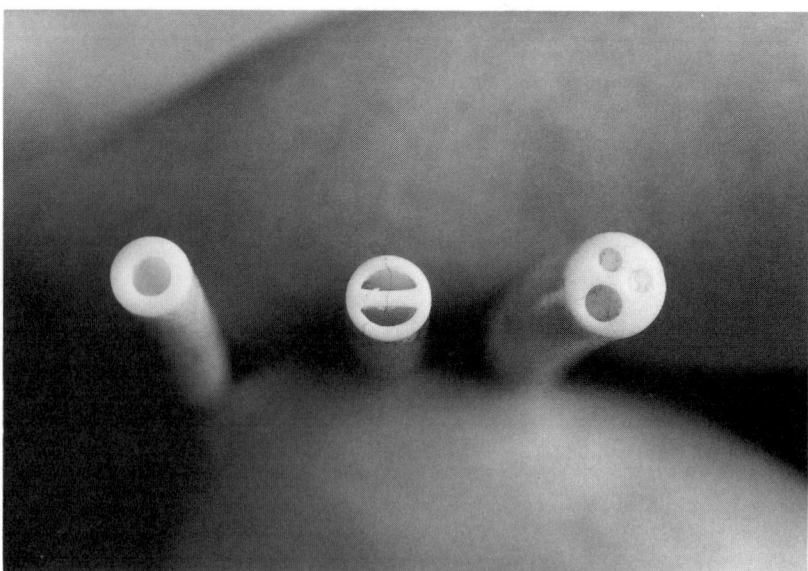

FIGURE 1-3. Configuration of the lumens of long-term venous access catheters. On the left is a 9.6-Fr single lumen catheter with a 1.6 mm internal diameter. In the middle is a 10-Fr dual-lumen catheter with a double-D configuration. Each lumen has a 1.3 mm internal diameter. On the right is a 12.5-Fr triple-lumen Hickman catheter. The smaller lumens have a 1.0 mm internal diameter whereas that of the larger lumen is 1.3 mm. Note the thinner wall of the dual-lumen catheter which is possible because of the higher silicone content and slightly stiffer nature of the device.

stiffer to allow for larger lumens in a smaller diameter catheter. The triple-lumen 12.5-Fr Hickman catheter incorporates "two Broviacs and a Hickman" and is used primarily for bone marrow transplantation patients (Figure 1-4).

The Groshong catheter is an external device that is gaining in popularity and is distinguished by its modified slit-valve tip (Figure 1-5). The catheter provides an additional element of safety, convenience, and cost efficiency. The slit valve alongside the tip is designed to minimize the possibility of catheter lumen occlusion caused by passive reflux of blood into the lumen and to reduce the need for daily heparin flushing (Figure 1-6). At present the manufacturer's recommendation for Groshong catheters is to flush weekly with non-heparinized saline. One study, however, has reported that clots frequently could be aspirated from the lumens of Groshong catheters in cancer patients,[5] suggesting that the reflux of blood into the lumens is not completely prevented by the slit-valve design. These features of the Groshong catheter potentially represent a substantial reduction in the maintenance requirements and cost to the patient. In contrast to the Hickman catheter, the Groshong catheter is inserted and positioned in the vein initially and then tunneled to an exit site on the

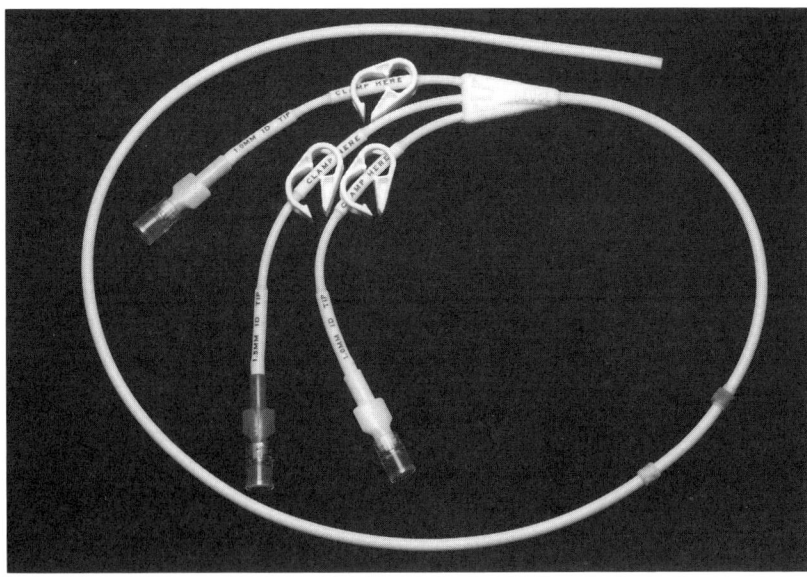

FIGURE 1-4. Triple-lumen 12.5-Fr Hickman catheter.

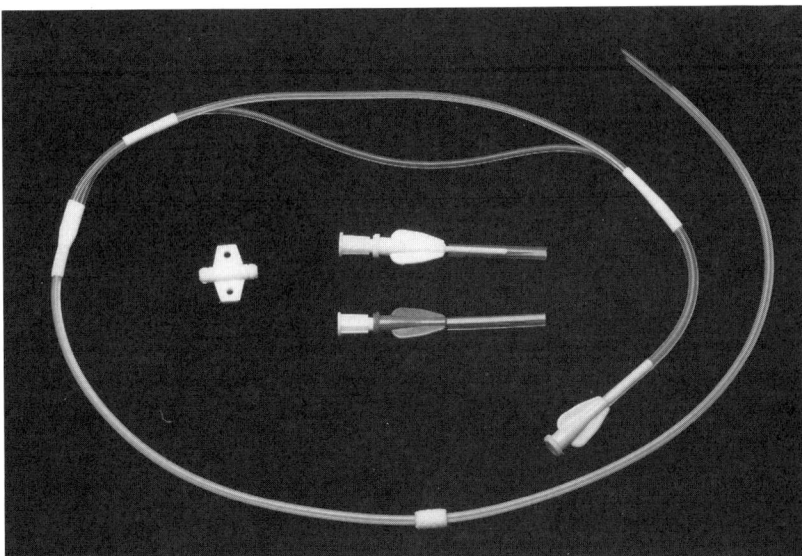

FIGURE 1-5. Dual-lumen Groshong catheter. The slit-valve tip is initially placed in its appropriate location within the vein. The remainder of the catheter is then tunneled subcutaneously through an exit site on the precordium. The end of the catheter is then cut to provide two separate catheter access lumens and the external hubs are then secured to the cut ends of the catheter. Note that no external clamps are required in the catheter design.

8 Vascular Access in the Cancer Patient

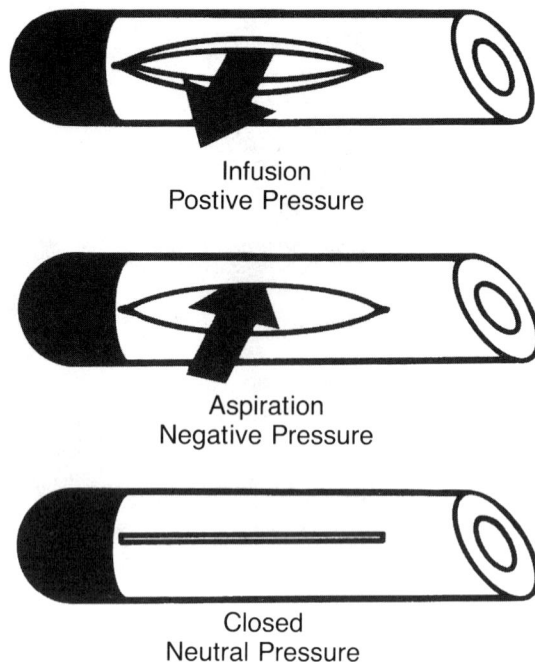

FIGURE 1-6. Schematic illustration of the Groshong catheter tip. The slit along the side of the catheter remains closed when the catheter is not in use and prevents passive reflux of blood into the lumen. The slit along the side of the catheter near the tip allows for aspiration of blood products and infusion of fluids in response to negative or positive pressure.

precordium. The catheter is then cut to length and coupled to the external hubs. The Groshong is also available as a single 3.5-, 5.5-, 7-, and 8-Fr, or double, 5- and 9.5-Fr, lumen catheter. The Groshong is a thin-walled Silastic catheter so that in general the smaller French sizes provide a lumen diameter comparable to those larger Hickman sizes. For instance, the 8-Fr Groshong catheter provides the same internal diameter lumen as the 9.6-Fr Hickman.

External devices are available as percutaneous insertion kits with guidewire, dilator, peel-away sheath, tunneler, syringes, needles, and caps included (Figure 1-7).

Implantable Ports

Implantable ports are constructed of plastic or titanium and have a silicone diaphragm (Figure 1–8). The housing is designed to be biocompatible, durable, have low thrombogenicity, and produce minimal computed tomography (CT) or magnetic resonance imaging (MRI) image distortion. The port comes either preconnected to the catheter or is attachable to the catheter at the time of insertion with a

Long-Term Venous Access Catheters and Implantable Ports 9

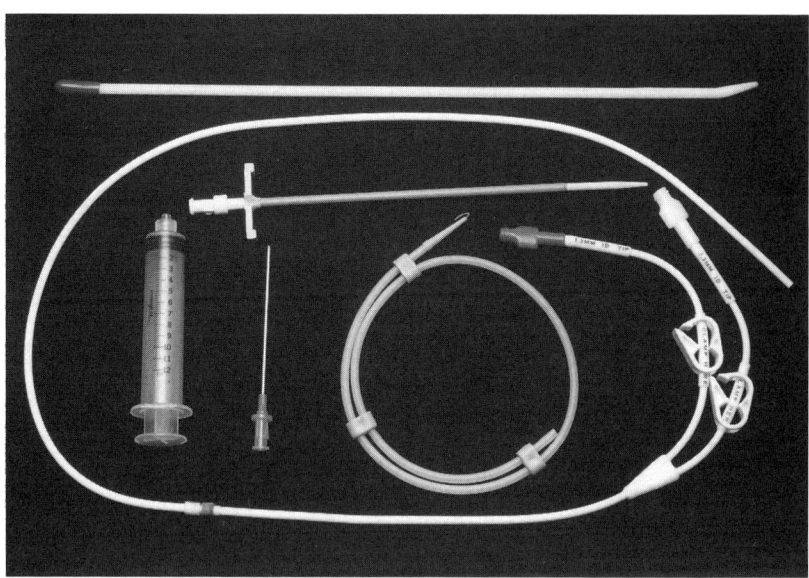

FIGURE 1-7. Long-term venous access catheter insertion kit includes a catheter, syringe and needle for venapuncture, J-wire for venous cannulation, a vessel dilator/peel away sheath complex for catheter insertion, and a plastic trocar for creation of a subcutaneous tunnel.

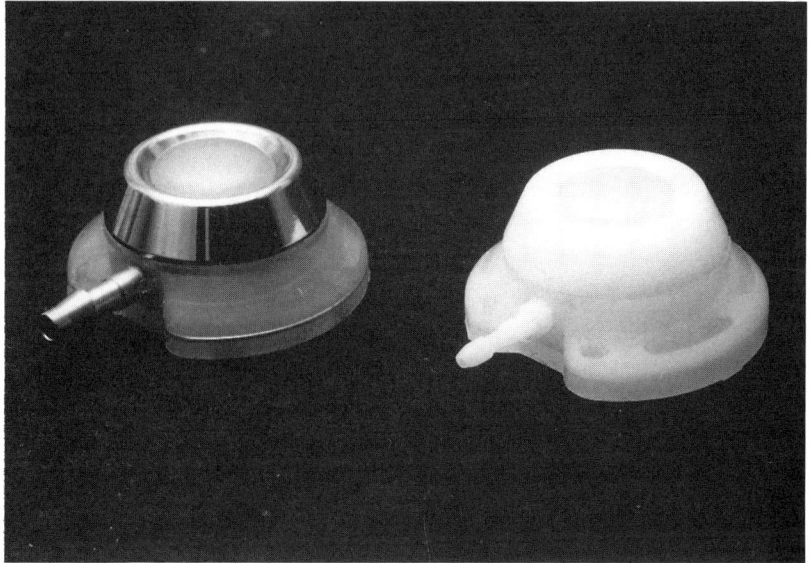

FIGURE 1-8. Implantable port housings constructed of titanium (*left*) or plastic (*right*). Note the silicone diaphragm for venous access with a noncoring needle.

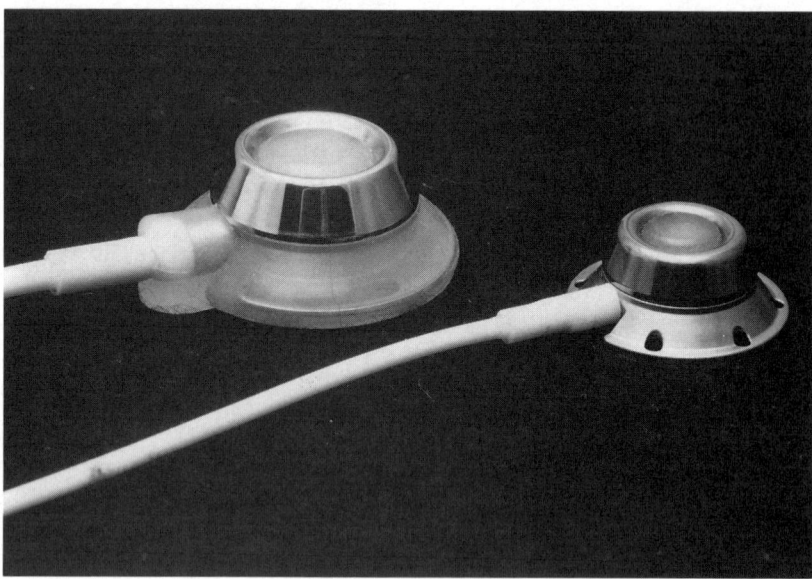

FIGURE 1-9. Standard adult implantable port housing (*left*) compared to the "low-profile" implantable port housing for pediatric or very thin adult patients (*right*).

sleeve or other type of locking mechanism. In addition, a single-lumen smaller implantable port or "low-profile" device is available to accommodate pediatric or very thin adult patients (Figure 1-9). A double-lumen implantable port is also available (Figure 1-10). The septum of the port housing is made of compressed silicone to provide optimum needle stability and retention, and to protect against extravasation, and is designed to withstand multiple punctures with a noncoring needle. An implantable port housing with a dome-shaped silicone access port is available (Figure 1-11). The adult-sized device (9.6-Fr) has a 2.8 mm outside and 1.6 mm inside diameter. The port housing is approximately 1 cm across and has a height of 13.5 mm whereas the low-profile port is 10.1 mm high and is available with a 6.6-Fr catheter. The dual-lumen port housing is larger, with base dimensions of 26.7 × 16.5 mm. The catheter that attaches to the dual-lumen port housing is either a 9.5-Fr Groshong or 10-Fr or 12-Fr Hickman. The double-lumen ports with attachable catheters have staggered lumens at the tip to prevent infusate precipitation.

Strum prospectively evaluated the clinical performance of implantable ports with either a small bore (0.51 mm) or large-bore (1.02 mm) internal diameter.[6] Overall, there was an occlusion rate of 21.5% (7 of 32 catheters); however, occlusions occurred only in patients with small-bore catheters (7 of 16, 44%) despite the use of

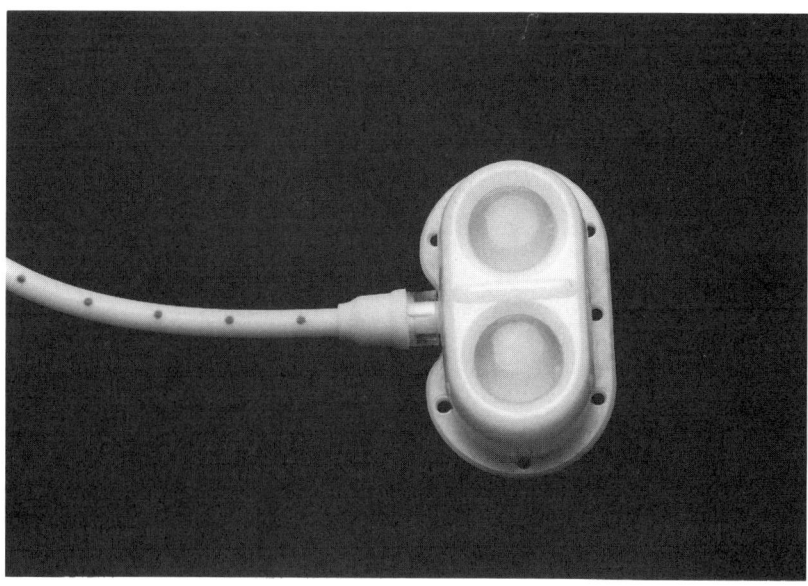

FIGURE 1-10. Dual-lumen plastic implantable port housing.

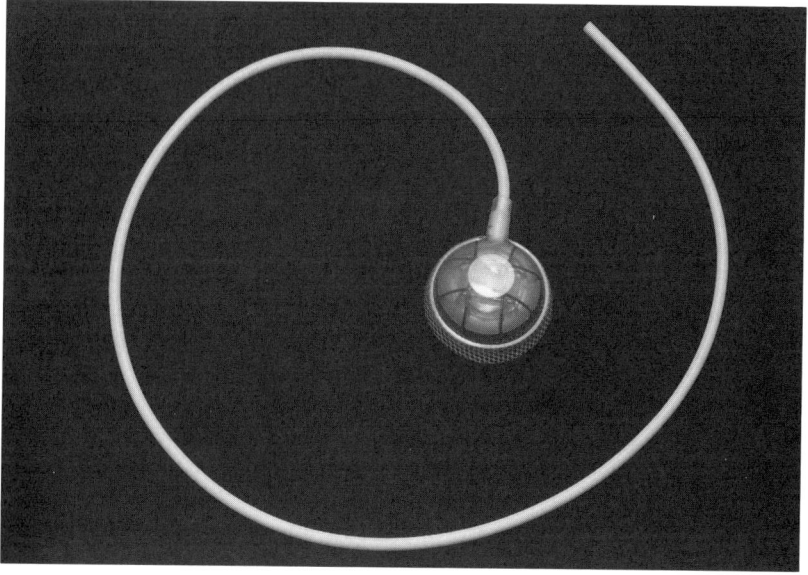

FIGURE 1-11. Dome-shaped implantable port housing. (Omega-port, Norfolk, VA.)

12 *Vascular Access in the Cancer Patient*

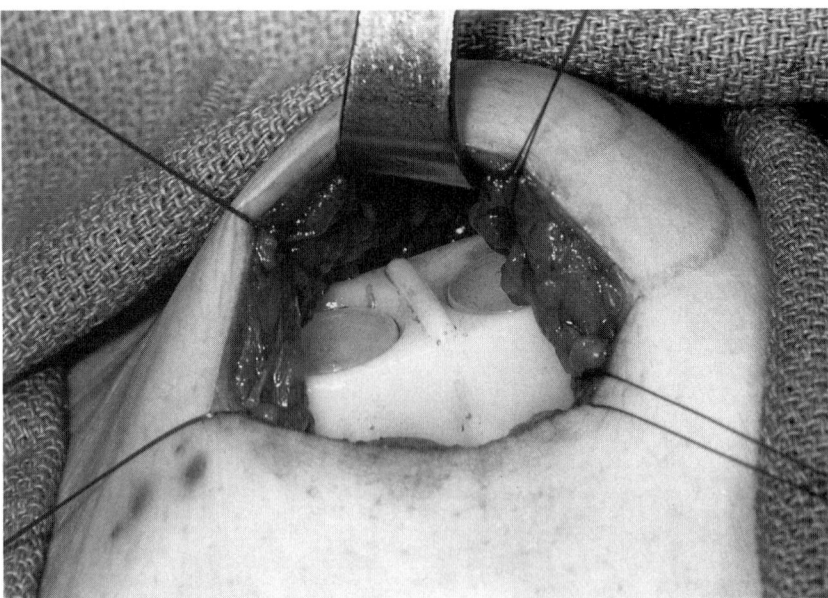

FIGURE 1-12. Implantable port housing anchored in four quadrants to underlying fascia to prevent malpositioning.

continuous infusion therapy. This would suggest that the routine use of the commercially available adult-sized devices is preferable for most patients and that smaller bore devices should be reserved for pediatric patients.

Ports are placed into subcutaneous pockets and when the catheter is inserted into the subclavian, external jugular, or internal jugular vein, the port is anchored to the pectoralis fascia on the anterior chest wall. All ports have suture holes or a silicone cuff at the base of the housing so that they can be secured to the underlying fascia which will eliminate the possibility of the port flipping over within the pocket (Figure 1-12).

Ports are accessed with a noncoring Huber point needle to minimize the possibility of damage to the septum (Figure 1-13). The needles are available as either straight or bent at a 90° angle, in various gauges and lengths. The 90° bent needle provides a low-profile access to the port and minimizes the chance of inadvertent dislodgement. Because the septum on the port housing must be palpated to gain access, ports should not be placed in deep subcutaneous pockets and are not ideally suited for patients who are obese.

Like the external devices, ports are available with an introducer set which includes guidewire, dilator, peel away sheath, needles, syringes, and noncoring needle.

Other Types of CVCs

Generally thought of as short-term, percutaneous CVCs have been in use in hospitals for many decades and are intended to be placed for periods of days to several weeks. Often used for postoperative management or other acute care needs, they may be single- or multi-lumen and are composed of silicone or polyurethane. Advantages of these CVCs over the surgically placed semipermanent devices include bedside placement, cost savings, and ease of removal, as well as the ability to use the same puncture site to change the catheter over a guidewire should a problem occur. Maintenance of these devices has been well defined, and in experienced hands morbidity should be no greater in the cancer patient than in the noncancer patient.

A critical reevaluation of nontunneled, noncuffed silastic CVCs as an alternative to tunneled or implanted devices for long-term venous access has been presented by Raad et al.[7] One hundred eighty-eight subclavian vein CVCs were placed in adult cancer patients for long-term venous access and maintained by an infusion team or by patients or family members trained in catheter care. With a mean duration of 136 days per catheter, the rate of infectious complications was extremely low compared to many series with tunneled long-term venous access catheters (Table 1-2). The risk of developing infectious complications was not associated with the use of steroids, neutropenia, renal insufficiency, thrombocytopenia, or history of bone marrow transplantation. Importantly, the estimated cost savings from the use of nontunneled CVCs were substantial compared to the calculated costs of inserting and maintaining the same number of tunneled long-term venous catheters. When one considers that a subclavian vein CVC can be placed in the clinic setting without the need for an

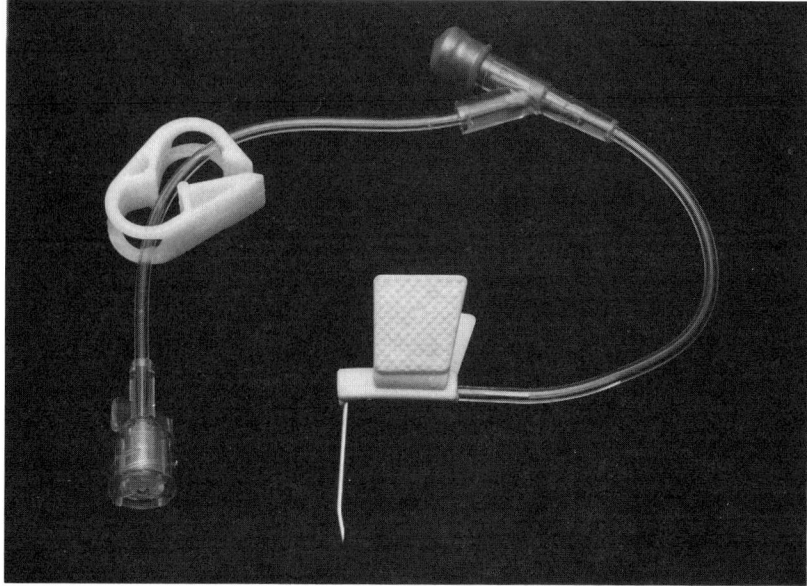

FIGURE 1-13. Noncoring Huber needle for implantable port access. Note the angled tip to prevent coring of the silicone septum and the 90° angulation of the needle to prevent inadvertent dislodgement.

TABLE 1-2
Rate of Infectious Complications in Nontunneled Long-Term Subclavian CVCs in Adult Cancer Patients

No. of catheters	188
Mean duration (days)	136
Exit site inflammation (%)	5 (2.7)
Catheter-related bacteremia (%)	5 (2.7)
Total infections/100 catheter use days	0.09

Modified from Raad I, Davis S, Becker M, et al. Low infection rate and long durability of nontunneled Silastic catheters. Arch Intern Med 1993;153:1791–1796.

anesthesiologist, operating room, or fluoroscopy, the cost of inserting and maintaining these CVCs on a monthly basis has been estimated to be approximately one fifth of that for tunneled catheters. In contrast to a tunneled long-term venous catheter, in the event of suspected line sepsis a nontunneled CVC can be changed over a guidewire for the purposes of diagnosis. The successful use of these CVCs in this setting attests to their safety and utility compared to tunneled long-term venous access devices. A more complete review of CVCs is presented in Chapter 8.

Repair Kits

Catheters are at risk for leaks or breaks in the external segment simply because they are manipulated so frequently. If a break occurs in either a single- or a multi-lumen catheter, it may be repaired with the appropriate repair kit (available from the manufacturer) by specially trained nurses or physicians if the break is distant enough from the exit site to allow the repair limb to be attached to an adequate length of old catheter. These catheters have different diameters, so repair kits are not interchangeable. Only the repair kit specifically designed for the type and diameter of the catheter should be used. Before a catheter is repaired, the exit site should be inspected for signs of inflammation or infection. If the skin around the exit site is normal or only minimally inflamed, the catheter may be repaired. The repair of any type of catheter is a sterile procedure. Some catheters, such as the Groshong, may be repaired using a simple replacement section that contains a stylet. After the damaged section of the catheter is removed, the replacement section is inserted into the remaining catheter, the stylet is withdrawn, and the replacement segment is snap-locked onto the catheter.

A much more cumbersome repair procedure is required for the Hickman-type catheters. The replacement section of the catheter has a permanent metal stylet and an external sleeve that slides over the repair site (Figure 1-14). In preparation for the repair, the replacement section is primed with heparin flush solution and a syringe with a

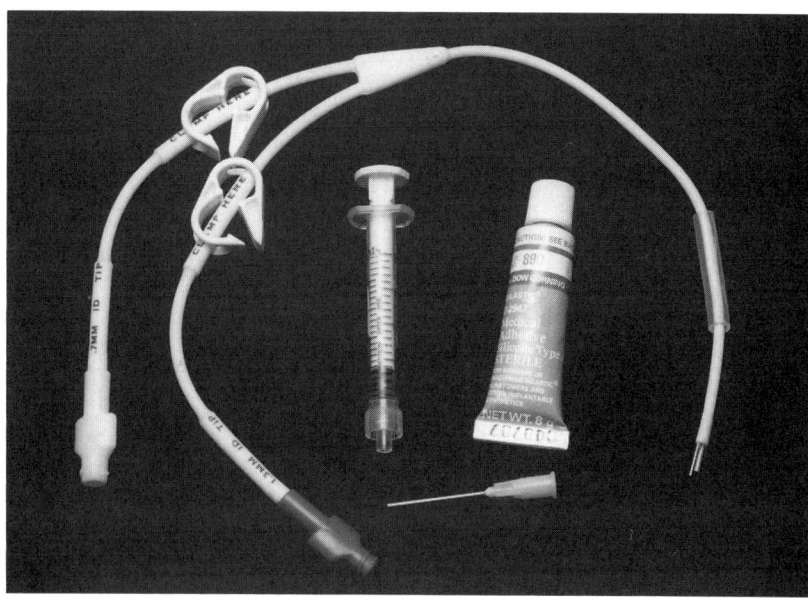

FIGURE 1-14. Components of the repair kit that is available for replacement of damaged or fractured external portions of long-term venous access catheters.

blunt needle is filled with silastic glue. After the damaged section of the catheter is removed, the metal stylet is inserted into the remaining catheter and silastic glue is applied over the repair site. The external sleeve is then slipped over the connection and more silastic glue is injected under both ends of the outer sleeve. Using a gauze pad, the outer sleeve is rolled around with the fingers to distribute the glue evenly. The repaired catheter may be used immediately; however, the connection site must be anchored with a tongue blade for 24 hours for support while the glue is drying.

References

1. Broviac JW, Cole JJ, Schribner BH. A silicone rubber atrial catheter for prolonged parenteral alimentation. Surg Gynecol Obstet 1973; 136:602–606.
2. Hickman RO, Buckner CD, Clife RA, Sanders JE, Stewart P, Thomas ED. A modified right atrial catheter for access to the venous system in marrow transplant recipients. Surg Gynecol Obstet 1979;148:871–875.
3. Wagman LD, Kirkemo A, Johnston MR. Venous access: a prospective, randomized study of the Hickman catheter. Surgery 1984;95:303–308.
4. Niederhuber JE, Ensminger W, Gyves JW, Lipeman M, Doan K,

Cozzi E. Totally implanted venous and arterial access system to replace external catheters in cancer treatment. Surgery 1982; 92:706–712.
5. Anderson AJ, Krasnow, SH, Boyer, MW, Wadleigh, RG, and Cohen, MH. Clots can frequently be aspirated from Groshong catheters. Am Assoc Cancer Res 1988;29:A907:228. (Abstract)
6. Strum S, McDermed J, Korn A, Joseph C. Improved methods for venous access: the Port-A-Cath, a totally implanted catheter system. J Clin Oncol 1986;4:596–603.
7. Raad I, Davis S, Becker M, et al. Low infection rate and long durability of nontunneled Silastic catheters. Arch Intern Med 1993;153:1791–1796.

2
Clinical Performance of Long-Term Venous Access Devices

H. Richard Alexander

Single- vs Double-Lumen Devices
Implanted Ports vs External Catheters
Ports vs External Catheters: Infectious and
 Thrombotic Complications
Ports vs External Catheters in Pediatric
 Oncology Patients
Ports vs External Catheters in Adult
 Cancer Patients
Conclusions
References

Both the external and implanted port catheters have unique features that make the selection of one type of device more appropriate for some patients and not others. In addition, there are unique problems that can occur with either device. Implanted ports can develop pocket infections, can be difficult to access, and ports have been reported to flip over in the subcutaneous pocket or erode through the skin with the catheter in situ (Figure 2-1). External catheters can fracture at an extracorporeal location or can be inadvertently dislodged particularly within the first 2 to 3 weeks after insertion. The ideal venous access catheter should provide long-term, low-complication access to the venous system with minimal risk during insertion or removal, ease of maintenance, low cost, and good patient acceptance.

The selection of an external catheter or implanted port and the decision to use a single- vs dual-lumen catheter depend on several factors including the anticipated intensity of treatment, need for close monitoring of blood samples, need for frequent transfusions or intravenous fluid resuscitation, and patient preference. For patients receiving bolus injections of chemotherapy as outpatients on an intermittent basis, the implanted port may be most suitable. Implanted ports are routinely flushed with dilute heparin solution monthly when not in use, do not require a bandage when not in use, and have minimal interference with lifestyle. Patients best suited for external catheters include those receiving (1) potentially toxic regimens given as prolonged continuous infusions, (2) frequent supplemental intra-

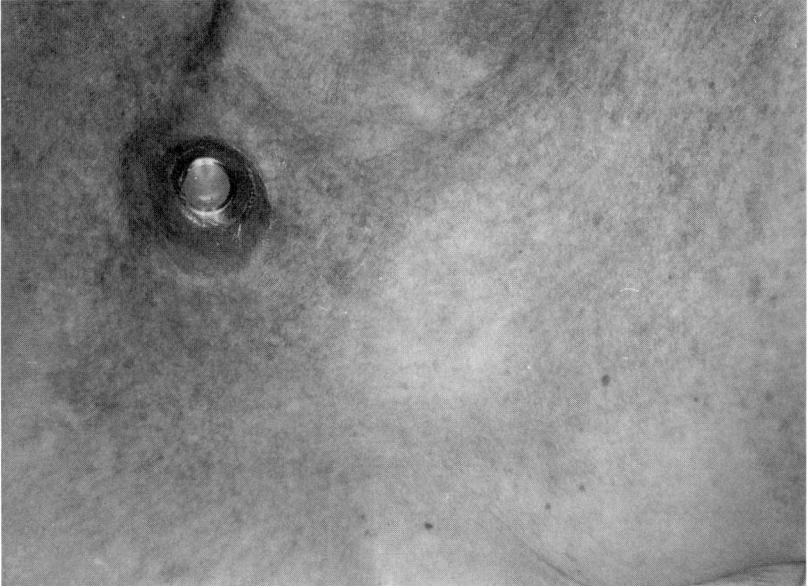

FIGURE 2-1. Implanted port housing that has eroded through the skin. (Courtesy of Alice B. Lucas, R.N., M.B.A., New York, NY.)

venous fluids or blood products, (3) frequent monitoring of blood counts, or (4) total parenteral nutrition.

Single- vs Double-Lumen Devices

Both external catheters and implanted ports are available as either single- or double-lumen catheters and the decision to use a double- vs a single-lumen device should be carefully weighed. Hayward et al reported very detailed follow-up of 100 patients with long-term venous access devices placed predominantly for chemotherapy.[1] Of the 22 catheters that were removed after completion of treatment, in 7 of the 12 double-lumen Hickman catheters only one lumen was used throughout the life of the catheter. Early et al retrospectively reviewed the outcomes of 51 single-lumen and 94 double-lumen Hickman catheters in adult cancer patients and compared them for types and frequency of complications necessitating catheter removal.[2] A higher infection rate was found with double-lumen catheters and the time to removal because of infectious complications was significantly shorter compared with single-lumen catheters (Table 2-1). However, there was no difference in the overall complication rate requiring removal of the catheter (Table 2-2). A prospective comparison of double- vs single-lumen external catheters reported by Haire et al showed that there was a marked trend for double lumen catheters to cause totally occlusive venous thrombosis more frequently than single-lumen catheters.[3] Thirty-nine percent of double-lumen catheters vs 8% of single-lumen catheters resulted in thrombi.

Implanted Ports vs External Catheters

A comparison of the major features of external catheters and implanted ports is presented in Table 2-3. Both devices can be inserted

TABLE 2-1
Relationship Between the Number of Catheter Lumens and the Rate and Time Course of Infectious Complications with Hickman Catheters

	Single-Lumen	Double-Lumen
No. of catheters	51	94
No. (%) of infected catheters	7 (14)	20 (21)
Infection rate, days in place	1/1210	1/496*
Time to infection (days)	213	78*

*$P \leq .02$ versus single-lumen.
Modified from Early TF, Gregory RT, Wheeler JR, Snyder SO Jr, Gayle RG. Increased infection rate in double-lumen versus single-lumen Hickman catheters in cancer patients. South Med J 1990;83:34–36.

TABLE 2-2
Relationship Between the Number of Lumens in Hickman Catheters and the Rate of Any Complication Requiring Removal

	Single-Lumen	Double-Lumen
No. of catheters	51	94
Longevity (mean, days)	116	106
Infection	7 (14%)	20 (21%)
Mechanical failure	7 (14%)	9 (10%)
Venous thrombosis	2 (4%)	2 (2%)
Total complication rate	31%	33%

Modified from Early TF, Gregory RT, Wheeler JR, Snyder SO Jr, Gayle RG. Increased infection rate in double-lumen versus single-lumen Hickman catheters in cancer patients. South Med J 1990;83:34–36.

while the patient is under a local anesthetic with monitored sedation. External catheters are easily removed in an office setting whereas the removal of an implanted port requires a second procedure. The implanted port is cosmetically superior as it lies under the skin and when not in use interferes minimally with lifestyle. Patient acceptance of implanted ports appears to be higher than that of external catheters and this has been well documented in the pediatric oncology population.[4] The external catheter does require routine maintenance such as cleaning of the exit site or daily flushing of the catheter lumens. When not in use, the port does not require any site care (other than normal hygiene) or bandage and most centers flush ports once a month when not in use. On the other hand, a port must be accessed with a Huber

TABLE 2-3
Comparison of the Features of External and Totally Implantable Venous Access Catheters

External Catheters	Implantable Ports
Double-lumen catheter easily inserted	Double-lumen available but port is large

Regular maintenance requirements
  Wound care
  Heparin flushing
	Minimal maintenance
	  No dressings
	  Monthly heparin flush

Restricts some activities such as swimming	Cosmetically superior, minimal interference with lifestyle, better patient acceptance
Maximal reliability for safe continuous intravenous therapy and blood sampling	Best suited for intermittent or maintenance chemotherapy; requires access with needle
Higher maintenance costs	Higher initial costs
Easy to remove	Requires second procedure to remove device

TABLE 2-4
*Relative Frequency of Complications Related to Totally Implantable Ports**

Complication	Percent
Arrhythmia	0.9
Arterial puncture	1.5
Embolism	0.6
Extravasation	6.4
Hematoma	1.8
Infection	
Local	15.2
Systemic	1.2
Migration	2.4
Pain	0.6
Pneumothorax	2.4
Skin necrosis	1.5
Thrombosis	
Catheter	9.1
Venous	4.9
Unable to insert	0.9
No complication	61.1

*Complications from 329 consecutively placed ports
Adapted from Brothers TE, Von Moll LK, Niederhuber JE, Roberts JA, Walker-Andrews S, Ensminger WD. Experience with subcutaneous infusion ports in three hundred patients. Surg Gynecol Obstet 1988;166:295–301.

needle each time it is used. This can produce substantial patient discomfort and requires that the needle be checked regularly to ensure that it has not dislodged. For infusional therapy over a long period of time, there is a risk that the access needle could dislodge and deliver drug or antibiotic subcutaneously. Brothers et al reported the experience at the University of Michigan with 329 implanted ports in place for a median of 257 days and found that extravasation secondary to the dislodgement of the Huber needle from the port diaphragm occurred in 6.4% of patients.[5] The other complications associated with insertion and use of the ports in this series are shown in Table 2-4. Interestingly, there was no increase in complications associated with using the port immediately after insertion. The ability to withdraw blood was documented in 188 ports and was always possible in 84% and intermittent in 11%.

    Initial costs of the implanted ports are higher than those of external devices. However, the cost of routine external catheter maintenance is higher so that after about 6 months of use the overall cost is about equal.[4,6] If the length of time required for venous access is substantially less than 6 months it may be more cost effective to consider an external device.

Ports vs External Catheters: Infectious and Thrombotic Complications

The most serious issues associated with long-term venous access are infectious and thrombotic complications and most studies comparing the two types of devices have focused on these issues (Table 2-5). Kappers-Klunne et al have reported a prospective randomized study evaluating the infectious complications associated with 20 implanted ports vs 23 catheters in adult patients with primarily hematological malignancies.[7] The overall infectious complication rate with double-lumen catheters vs implanted ports was comparable with 7 of 23 catheter-related infections and 4 of 20 port related. The duration of catheter use and number of days of granulocytopenia, or selective gut decontamination did not appear to correlate with the development of infection in either group. Carde et al have reported a prospective randomized trial of external catheters vs implanted ports in 100 adult patients with solid tumors.[8] Of the 81 patients alive at the end of the 6-month observation period significantly more patients had external catheters removed (20 of 39) than implanted ports (4 of 42). Of note, the most common reason for external catheter removal was "catheter fall" or accidental removal in six patients. An accidental catheter removal rate of 15% is high and accounts for the significant differences detected between the groups in this study. The infectious complication rate leading to catheter removal was also higher, although not significantly, with the external catheters (5 of 39, 12%) than with ports (1 of 40, 2.5%). Hayward et al have reported that the phenomenon of "falling out" occurs most commonly in patients with short, less than 6 cm, subcutaneous tunnels and in whom the cuff resides within 0.5 cm of the exit site, with the average, time to inadvertent removal being about 14 days after insertion.[1] Although adequate preoperative patient teaching may be the most important factor in minimizing the possibility of inadvertent catheter removal, this study does indicate that meticulous insertion technique with an adequate subcutaneous tunnel is important in minimizing the possibility of inadvertent removal.

Pegues et al have reported a retrospective matched cohort study in adult patients with solid tumors with external catheters or implanted ports.[9] This study compared the catheter related infection rates in 47 patients with Hickman catheters and 94 patients with implanted ports. Patients were matched for diagnosis, age, sex, presence of metastases, and date of insertion. The catheter-related infection rate was significantly higher with Hickman catheters than with ports, 1.8 vs 0.4 infections/1000 catheter use days, respectively. However, in this study patients with Hickman catheters had a significantly shorter survival and most patients with external catheters were receiving terminal hospice care at home compared to those with ports.

TABLE 2-5
Summary of Selected Reports Comparing the Performance of External Catheters vs Implanted Ports

Author	Patient	Diagnosis	Study	N H/B	N P	Median duration (d) H/B	Median duration (d) P	Patient Age H/B	Patient Age P	Complications H/B	Complications P	Parameter
Kappers-Klunne et al[7]	Adult	Leukemia	Prospective random	23	20	166	164	46	42	7/23	4/20	Infection[*]
Carde et al[8]	Adult	Solid tumors	Prospective random	46	50	—	—	49	49	20/39	4/42	All causes[†]
										5/39	1/40	Infection[†]
Pegues et al[9]	Adult	Solid tumors	Retrospective cohort	47	94	—	—	—	—	1.8	0.4	Infection[‡]
Guenier et al[10]	Adult	Various	Retrospective matched	148	299	69 (5–406)	233 (1–1298)	44	51	4.1	0.45	All causes[‡]
										41/144 (28%)	29/276 (10.5%)	All causes[§]
Hayward et al[1]	Adult	Various	Prospective nonrandom	71	29	—	—	—	—	21/71	4/29	All causes[11]
Shaw et al[11]	Adult	Various	Retrospective	61	39	70 (3–196)	168 (7–560)	23–88	17–74	66%	46%	Overall
										21%	3%	Sepsis
										33%	15%	Removals[§]
Greene et al[6]	Adult	Various	Retrospective	110	150	143	128	—	—	15%	3%	Sepsis
										22%	1%	Thrombosis
Ross et al[4]	Pediatric	Various	Prospective nonrandom	41	50	365	350	8	10	14/41	7/50	Overall°
										15/41	7/50	Infectious°
Mirro et al[14]	Pediatric	Mostly leukemic	Prospective	B: 113 H: 91	82	—	—	H: 12.3 B: 2.7	11.9	—	—	↑H/B failures° ↑H/B infection[++]
Ingram et al[16]	Pediatric	Various	Prospective nonrandom	130	144	116	166	3	8	16/130 (12%)	6/144 (4%)	Infection°
										14/130 (11%)	2/144 (1.4%)	Dislodgement°

H, Hickman; B, Broviac; P, port.
* $P = .66$, infection requiring early removal.
† $P < .001$, removal from all causes.
‡ Complication rate per 1000 catheter use days.
§ Number requiring early removal.
[11] $P < .1$, all complications leading to removal.
° $P < .002$.
** $P < .01$.

This would suggest that the patients in this study with Hickman catheters generally had more advanced disease, were more debilitated, and may have been predisposed to infectious complications. Guenier et al have reported a large retrospective study of 148 Hickman/Broviac catheters compared to 299 implanted ports (Port-A-Cath) in adult cancer patients with a variety of malignancies.[10] The average external catheter remained in situ for an average of 68.6 days and in 28% of patients was removed for a complication prior to the end of treatment. On the other hand, implanted ports remained in situ for an average of 232.9 days and were removed prior to completion of treatment in 10.5%. The overall complication rate was higher with external catheters compared to ports, 4.1 vs 0.45/1000 catheter days, respectively. Infection was the most common complication in either group and represented 78% of all complications with external catheters and 52% of all port-related complications. In this study, there was a substantial disparity in the diagnoses of patients with external catheters or implanted ports; approximately 80% of those receiving external catheters had hematological malignancies for which most underwent bone marrow transplantation. In contrast, almost 90% of patients with ports had breast cancer. This difference in the type of tumors between the two groups indicates that there may be other differences such as general medical condition, intensity of treatment, and degree of immunosuppression that could account in some part for the observed differences in catheter duration and infectious complications. Shaw et al have also reported a retrospective review of 100 consecutive catheter insertions of which 61 were external devices and 39 were implanted ports in adult cancer patients.[11] In this study as well, the majority of patients receiving Hickman catheters had leukemia whereas most patients receiving implanted ports had solid tumor malignancies. Despite the fact that the mean duration of insertion for ports was over twice as long as for external catheters, the incidence of overall complications was 66% for Hickman catheters and 46% for ports which were severe enough to warrant removal in 33% and 15%, respectively. Line-related septicemia occurred in 21% of Hickman catheters and in 3% of ports. Other complications including line fracture or kinking occurred rarely with either type of device.

In a retrospective review of adult patients matched for age, diagnosis, treatment, and nutritional status receiving either external or implanted ports, Greene et al[6] identified a higher incidence of infectious and thrombotic complications in patients with external catheters (15% and 22%, respectively) compared to patients with implanted ports (3% and 1% respectively). Of note, in the two groups catheters were inserted during two sequential time periods. The thrombotic complication rate associated with external catheters (22%) that were inserted several years earlier than the implanted ports is higher than in more recent studies[12] and may reflect on the progress in routine catheter maintenance that has developed with time.

Stanislav et al have compared the results of using 44 Hickman

TABLE 2-6
Complications Requiring Removal of External Catheters Are More Frequent Compared to Implanted Ports: Results of a Retrospective Study in Adults

	No. (%) of Patients	
	Catheters (N = 44)	Ports (N = 71)
Catheter-related complications		
Infection	7 (16)	8 (11)
Thrombosis	5 (11)	4 (6)
Miscellaneous	5 (11)	1 (1)
Total complications	17 (38)	13 (18)*
Complication rate (days)	1/501	1/1450†

*$P < .03$.
†$P < .005$.
Modified from Stanislav GV, Fitzgibbons RJ Jr, Bailey RT Jr, Malliard JA, Johnson S, Feole JB. Reliability of implantable central venous access devices in patients with cancer. Arch Surg 1991;122:1280–1283.

catheters and 71 implanted ports in adult cancer patients.[13] Although there was no difference in the rate of infectious or thrombotic complications between the two types of devices, the total number of complications and overall complication rates were significantly lower with implanted ports (Table 2-6). Of note, although the frequency of catheter related venous thrombosis was not related to catheter type it did appear to correlate with the position of the catheter tip. The incidence of venous thrombosis increased with catheter tips located high in the superior vena cava or above whereas there were no catheter related venous thromboses when the catheter tip was located in the low superior vena cava or the right atrium (Table 2-7).

Ports vs External Catheters in Pediatric Oncology Patients

Ross et al have reported a prospective nonrandomized study comparing the complications, patient and parental acceptance, and costs in

TABLE 2-7
Relationship Between Catheter Tip Position and the Frequency of Thrombosis

Position	No. of Catheters	No. of Thromboses
Right atrium	31	0
Low superior vena cava	19	0
High superior vena cava	44	2
Above superior vena cava	19	6

Modified from Stanislav GV, Fitzgibbons RJ Jr, Bailey RT Jr, Maillard JA, Johnson S, Feole JB. Reliability of implantable central venous access devices in patients with cancer. Arch Surg 1991;122:1280–1283.

TABLE 2-8
Greater Acceptance of Implanted Ports vs External Venous Access Devices in Pediatric and Young Adult Patients

	Response (%)			
	Positive		Negative	
	Ports	Catheters	Ports	Catheters
Ease of care, all patients	94	57	6	43*
Comfort, all patients	80	73	20	27
Overall acceptance, all patients	80	75	15	16
>11 yrs	83	40*	8	20
<11 yrs	75	80	24	15

*$P < .001$.
Modified from Ross MN, Haase GM, Poole MA, Burrington JD, Odom LF. Comparison of totally implanted reservoirs with external catheters as venous access devices in pediatric oncologic patients. Surg Gynecol Obstet 1988;167:141–144.

pediatric oncology patients receiving catheters or ports.[4] Most patients had a diagnosis of leukemia or lymphoma and were comparably distributed between patients receiving either type of catheter. Overall and infectious complications were significantly higher with external catheters compared to ports (Table 2-5). Child and parental surveys showed that ports were easier to care for and more readily accepted by children greater than 11 years of age (Table 2-8). Mirro et al, in another prospectively conducted study, evaluated the complications of Hickman, Broviac, and implanted ports in pediatric oncology patients.[14] Overall, there was a significantly higher failure-free duration of use with ports compared to either Hickman or Broviac type (Figure 2-2). In this study there was a clear difference in patient age and other clinical parameters in those receiving Broviac vs Hickman or ports. However, when Hickman catheters and ports were compared in clinically similar pediatric patients, there was a trend for lower infection rates in ports vs catheters. In a subset analysis of patients matched for diagnosis, intensity of therapy, and remission status (patients receiving Broviacs were still significantly younger), the failure-free interval was longer for ports vs Hickman catheters but not for implanted ports vs Broviac catheters. Similarly, the infection-free duration was longer, but not significantly, with ports vs catheters. When devices were used for longer than 400 days the infection rates became significantly lower with ports.

La Quaglia et al have reported the results of a prospective analysis of factors affecting the rates of infections in over 250 pediatric cancer patients with either external devices or implanted ports.[15] Table 2-9 shows the characteristics of the two populations and the differences in infection rates between the two groups. Of note, the patients who received external catheters were slightly younger than those

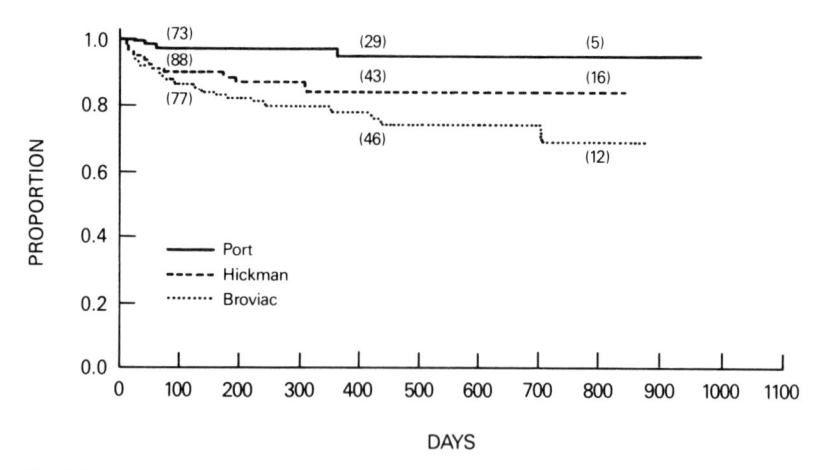

FIGURE 2-2. Time to catheter removal (for any complication including dislodgement, infection, or obstruction) in pediatric oncology patients with implantable ports, Hickman catheters, or Broviac catheters. The numbers in parentheses represent the number of patients analyzed at each time point. There was a significantly longer failure-free duration with implantable ports compared with external long-term venous access devices. Reproduced from Mirro JJ, Rao BN, Stokes DC, et al. A prospective study of Hickman/Broviac catheters and implantable ports in pediatric oncology patients. J Clin Oncol 1989;7:214–222.

receiving ports and the rate of infection and the proportion of devices removed secondary to infection were higher in patients with external devices. The time course to first infection in each group is illustrated in Figure 2-3. On the basis of multivariate analysis, patient age of less than 7 years and use of external catheters were associated with significantly higher infection rates than implanted ports and age greater than 7 years (Table 2-10).

In another study of pediatric oncology patients, Ingram et al have presented a prospective analysis of clinical and infectious complica-

TABLE 2-9

Results of a Prospective Comparison of Infectious Complications in Pediatric Oncology Patients with Either External Catheters or Implanted Ports

Parameter	External Catheters	Implanted Ports	P-Value
N	229	42	
Age (years)	72 ± 4.7	9.5 ± 4.8	<.01
Days in situ (median)	192	428	<.001
No. of infections	113 (49%)	9 (21%)	<.01
Removed (infection)	61 (30%)	5 (15%)	=.04

Modified from La Quaglia MP, Lucas A, Thaler HT, Friedlander-Klar H, Exelby PR, Groeger JS. A prospective analysis of vascular access device-related infections in children. J Pediatr Surg 1992;27:840–842.

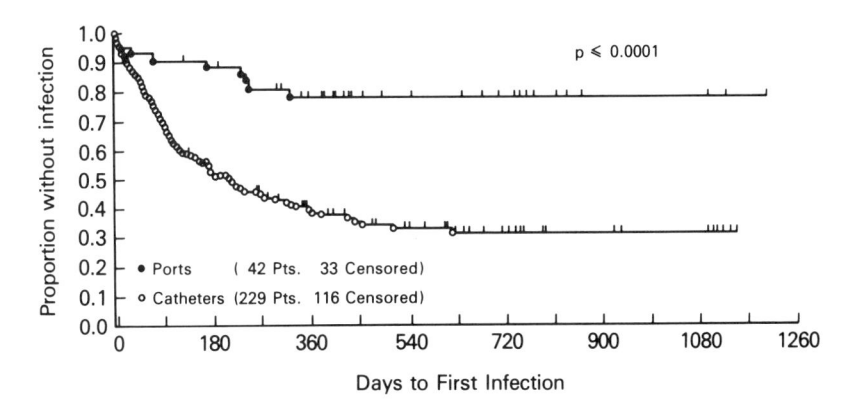

FIGURE 2-3. Time to first infection in pediatric patients with external catheters vs implanted ports. Patients with external catheters were twice as likely to develop infection (*P*<.0001). Reproduced from La Quaglia MP, Lucas A, Thaler HT, Friedlander-Klar H, Exelby PR, Groeger JS. A prospective analysis of vascular access device-related infections in children. J Pediatr Surg 1992;27:840–842. Used with permission.

tions of 144 consecutive implanted ports and 130 external catheters.[16] Overall, children receiving implanted ports were older than those receiving external catheters and there was an uneven distribution of disease categories between the groups. However, when patients were analyzed by age and diagnosis there was still a significantly higher incidence of infectious complications with external catheters compared to implanted ports. The indications for device removal in this series are presented in Table 2-11.

In contrast, Wurzel et al have observed comparable infections rates in pediatric oncology patients who had undergone placement of either an external device or an implanted port.[17] The patients were

TABLE 2-10
Results of a Multivariate Analysis of Factors Associated with Developing an Infectious Complication in Pediatric Oncology Patients with External Catheters or Implanted Ports

Parameter	Relative Risk Ratio	P-Value
Device type (catheter vs port)	1.96	≤.0001
Age (years) (≤ 7 vs > 7)	1.24	≤.002
Tumor type*	—	=.14

*Lymphomas, solid tumors, leukemia.
Modified from La Quaglia MP, Lucas A, Thaler HT, Friedlander-Klar H, Exelby PR, Groeger JS. A prospective analysis of vascular access device-related infections in children. J Pediatr Surg 1992;27:840–842.

TABLE 2-11
Indications for Removal of External Catheters or Ports in Pediatric Oncology Patients

	Catheters	Ports	P-Value
Total devices removed	101 (78%)	46 (32%)	<.0001
Treatment completed	29 (22%)	21 (15%)	NS
Patient choice	9 (7%)	0 (0%)	<.004
Death	22 (17%)	11 (8%)	<.03
Persistent infection	16 (12%)	6 (4%)	<.02
Blood	13 (10%)	1 (0.7%)	<.001
Pocket or tunnel	3 (2%)	5 (3%)	NS
Catheter occlusion	8 (6%)	2 (1.4%)	NS
Inadvertent catheter/needle dislodgement	14 (11%)	2 (1.4%)	<.002
Drug infiltration	0 (0%)	1 (0.7%)	NS
Mechanical occlusion/placement	2 (2%)	1 (0.7%)	NS
Catheter rupture (irreparable)	1 (1%)	2 (1.4%)	NS

NS, not significant.
Modified from Ingram J, Weitzman S, Greenberg ML, Parkin P, Filler R. Complications of indwelling venous access lines in the pediatric hematology patient: a prospective comparison of external venous catheters and subcutaneous ports. Am J Pediatr Hematol Oncol 1991;13:130–136.

well matched for age, gender, diagnosis, and use of perioperative antibiotics and were comparable with respect to the amount of time that they were neutropenic or hospitalized. In addition, the mean duration that the vascular access devices were in place and the percentage of time that they were accessed were equal. The infection rate was 0.21 per 100 catheter use days for external catheters and 0.14 per 100 catheter use days for implanted devices; the relative risk of infection in the external catheters was 1.5 compared to implanted devices, which was not significant. This study did demonstrate an association between age and tumor type and the risk of developing infection regardless of the type of vascular access device used (Table 2-12). Children less than 2 years of age were at higher risk for the development of infection compared to older children with either catheter type and the relative risk of infection in children less than 2 years was higher with external devices than with implanted ports. For children between 2 and 10 years of age the relative risk of infection was the same with either type of device but for children over 10 the relative risk with external devices was significantly lower than with implantable devices. In a multivariate analysis the percent of time with neutropenia correlated with the risk of developing infection and, again, this risk was highest in children less than 2 years old.

TABLE 2-12
Effect of Age and Tumor Type on the Relative Risk of Developing Catheter-Related Infection in Pediatric Oncology Patients with Either External Catheters (EC, N = 33) or Implanted Ports (IP, N = 45)

Parameter	Infection Rate/ 100 Catheter Days	Relative Risk (95% Confidence Interval)
EC		
Age (years)		
< 2	1.09	1.00
2–10	0.11	0.10 (0.04–0.31)
> 10	0	. . . (0.0–0.53)
<2 vs ≥ 2	—	0.08 (0.03–0.24)
Tumor type		
Leukemia	0.18	1.00
Solid	0.24	1.28 (0.45–3.70)
IP		
Age (years)		
< 2	0.49	1.00
2–10	0.10	0.21 (0.05–0.83)
> 10	0.15	0.31 (0.07–1.38)
<2 vs ≥ 2	—	0.24 (0.07–0.86)
Tumor type		
Leukemia	0.26	1.00
Solid	0.04	0.5 (0.03–0.70)

Modified from Wurzel CL, Halom K, Feldman JG, Rubin LG. Infection rates of Broviac-Hickman catheters and implantable venous devices. AJDC 1991;142:536–540.

Wiener et al, reporting the results of a prospective study conducted by the Children's Cancer Study Group (CCSG), did not find any difference in rates of removal secondary to infectious complications between external devices and implanted ports.[18] This large multiinstitutional study evaluated patient characteristics such as age and diagnosis, catheter types, insertion techniques, complications, function, and durability of external vs implanted vascular access devices. Of 1141 devices inserted in 1019 children there was follow-up on more than 95% of devices removed. At the time of analysis approximately two thirds of the vascular access devices had been removed. Significantly more implanted ports were removed electively than external catheters (Table 2-13). There were significantly more dislodgments of external catheters than implanted ports and, among external catheters, there were significantly more dislodgments with the smaller lumen devices. Dislodgments were associated with placement of the cuff within 2 cm of the exit site and in younger children (less than 3 years). There was no difference between external catheters and implanted ports with regard to removal rates attributable to infection.

TABLE 2-13
Results of a CCSG Prospective Study Comparing Causes for Removal of External Catheters (EC) vs Implanted Ports (IP) in Pediatric Cancer Patients

Parameter	Type of Catheter	
	EC	IP
N	735	290
Days per device (mean)	502	635
Percent removed		
Electively*	50%†	73%
Infection	19%	16%
Occlusion	4%	3%
Dislodgment	13%†	4%

*Electively defined as at the end of therapy or death.
†Significantly different than IP.
Modified from Weiner ES, McGuire P, Stolar CJH, et al. The CCSG prospective study of venous access devices: an analysis of insertions and causes for removal. J Pediatr Surg 1992;27:155–164.

Ports vs External Catheters in Adult Cancer Patients

The largest series comparing the clinical performance of Hickman vs implanted ports in adults come from the Memorial Sloan-Kettering Cancer Center. In an older review, Raaf et al presented clinical experience with a variety of vascular access techniques including arteriovenous grafts, various external catheters, and implanted ports and confirmed the reliability of Silastic catheters as a safe alternative to the more involved arteriovenous grafts.[19] More recently Groeger et al have presented a more detailed analysis of experience with 923 catheters and 707 implanted ports inserted over a 2-year period.[12] The decision to use ports vs external catheters in this series was based on clinical criteria and all catheters were followed prospectively for complications. Patients who received ports were older and had predominantly solid tumors whereas external catheters were inserted for patients with hematologic malignancies, bone marrow transplant, and childhood malignancies. With a minimum follow-up of 500 days the duration of function was longer with ports than with catheters (Table 2-14). More catheters were removed because of infection, catheter migration, death of the patient, and end of therapy than were ports (Table 2-15). Of note, the incidences of catheter lumen occlusion, catheter-related venous thrombosis, and persistent withdrawal occlusion were very low, about 1% or less, and similar for both types of devices. One retrospective review of more than 1422 venous access devices did demonstrate that a greater percentage of implanted ports

TABLE 2-14
Longevity of External Catheters and Implantable Ports in Cancer Patients

	Catheters	Ports
No. inserted	923	707
Male/female*	539/384	282/425
Age (years)*	28 ± 21 (26)	49 ± 18 (52)
Device days*	190,011	287,434
Days in situ*	205 ± 237 (125)	406 ± 307 (407)
Still in situ(%)*	62 (7)	179 (25)

*$P \leq .0001$ catheters vs ports.
Modified from Groeger JS, Lucas AB, Coit D. Venous access in the cancer patient. PPO Updates 1991;5:1–14.

were removed, primarily for malfunction, than external catheters.[20] However, as in other series, the rate of early overall venous access device removal because of malfunction or infection was very low, about 4%. These data illustrate the ability to prevent complications with an aggressive program of routine maintenance and catheter care.

May and Davis have compiled the results of all published literature that reported on infectious complications with vascular access catheters.[21] Pooled data indicated that external catheter life varied from a mean of 28 to 197 days. Infection rate varied from 8% to 80% and sepsis resulting in removal of the device occurred in 0 to 26% of cases. For implantable ports the infection rates were from 0 to 35% and sepsis necessitating removal occurred in 0 to 13% of cases. Overall the pooled data showed an infection rate per 100 days of 0.21 for external catheters and 0.4 for ports. It should be appreciated that all the studies pooled in this report indicate considerable variability in patient characteristics, diagnoses, indications for venous access, and

TABLE 2-15
Reasons for Catheter or Port Removal in Cancer Patients

	Catheters (%)	Ports (%)
No. removed*	861 (93)	528 (75)
End of therapy*	243 (26)	66 (9)
Death*	261 (28)	383 (54)
Infection*	229 (25)	34 (5)
Vessel thrombosis	10 (1)	7 (1)
Device clot	8 (0.8)	1 (0.1)
Infuses/no blood return	9 (1)	1 (0.1)
Tip migration/device extrusion*	65 (7)	3 (0.4)
Miscellaneous/other	36 (4)	33 (5)

*$P \leq .0001$ catheters vs ports.
Modified from Groeger JS, Lucas AB, Coit D. Venous access in the cancer patient. PPO Updates 1991;5:1–14.

criteria for diagnosing catheter-related infections. In addition, there is very likely to be considerable variability in the indications for catheter removal in different patient populations, different time periods, and among different institutions.

Conclusions

The preponderance of data appears to indicate that there are fewer infectious complications associated with ports than with external catheters. However, it also appears that in many studies the patient populations receiving external catheters or implanted ports are not well matched with respect to diagnosis, overall clinical condition, or intensity of treatment. As strict maintenance protocols and patient education programs become more uniformly adopted, the differences in reported infection rates may diminish. There is no consistent indication that the incidences of thrombotic or other complications are different with either device. However, it is also clear that the proven reliability and safety of external catheters have made them the preferred device for patients requiring intensive prolonged chemotherapy. This is particularly true for patients with hematological malignancies and those undergoing bone marrow transplantation. The external catheters can be used for intravenous resuscitation whereas the ports, typically accessed with a 20- or 22-gauge needle, may not be ideally suited for patients with frequent transfusion requirements or complex treatment requiring the availability of two lumens. Because many patients with dual-lumen catheters may actually use only one lumen through the life of the catheter and the incidence of infection may be greater with a dual-lumen catheter, the need for a single- vs double-lumen catheter should be carefully assessed. The implanted port appears best suited for those patients undergoing intermittent or maintenance chemotherapy.

References

1. Hayward SR, Ledgerwood AM, Lucas CE. The fate of 100 prolonged venous access devices. Am Surg 1990;56:515–519.
2. Early TF, Gregory RT, Wheeler JR, Snyder SO, Jr, Gayle RG. Increased infection rate in double-lumen versus single-lumen Hickman catheters in cancer patients. South Med J 1990;83:34–36.
3. Haire WD, Lieberman RP, Lund GB, Edney JA, Kessinger A, Armitage JO. Thrombotic complications of silicone rubber catheters during autologous marrow peripheral stem cell transplantation: prospective comparison of Hickman and Groshong catheters. Bone Marrow Transplant 1991;7:57–59.
4. Ross MN, Haase GM, Poole MA, Burrington JD, Odom LF. Comparison of totally implanted reservoirs with external catheters as venous access devices in pediatric oncologic patients. Surg Gynecol Obstet 1988;167:141–144.

5. Brothers TE, Von Moll LK, Niederhuber JE, Roberts JA, Walkerrews S, Ensminger WD. Experience with subcutaneous infusion ports in three hundred patients. Surg Gynecol Obstet 1988; 166:295–301.
6. Greene FL, Moore W, Strickl G, McFarl J. Comparison of a totally implantable access device for chemotherapy (Port-A-Cath) and long-term percutaneous catheterization (Broviac). South Med J 1988;81:580–603.
7. Kappers-Klunne MC, Degener JE, Stijnen T, Abels J. Complications from long-term indwelling central venous catheters in hematologic patients with special reference to infection. Cancer 1989;64:1747–1752.
8. Carde P, Cosset-Delaigue MF, LaPlanche A, Chareau I. Classical external indwelling central venous catheter versus totally implanted venous access systems for chemotherapy administration: a randomized trial in 100 patients with solid tumors. Eur J Cancer Clin Oncol 1989;25:939–944.
9. Pegues D, Axelrod P, McClarren C, et al. Comparison of infections in Hickman and implanted port catheters in adult solid tumor patients. J Surg Oncol 1992;49:156–162.
10. Guenier C, Ferreira J, Pector JC. Prolonged venous access in cancer patients. Eur J Surg Oncol 1989;15:553–555.
11. Shaw JHF, Douglas R, Wilson T. Clinical performance of Hickman and Portacath atrial catheters. Aust N Z J Surg 1988;58:657–659.
12. Groeger JS, Lucas AB, Coit D. Venous access in the cancer patient. PPO updates, 1991;5:1–14.
13. Stanislav GV, Fitzgibbons RJ, Jr, Bailey RT, Jr, Mailliard JA, Johnson S, Feole JB. Reliability of implantable central venous access devices in patients with cancer. Arch Surg 1991;122:1280–1283.
14. Mirro J, Jr, Rao BN, Stokes DC, et al. A prospective study of Hickman/Broviac catheters and implantable ports in pediatric oncology patients. J Clin Oncol 1989;7:214–222.
15. La Quaglia MP, Lucas A, Thaler HT, Friedler-Klar H, Exelby PR, Groeger JS. A prospective analysis of vascular access device-related infections in children. J Pediatr Surg 1992;27:840–842.
16. Ingram J, Weitzman S, Greenberg ML, Parkin P, Filler R. Complications of indwelling venous access lines in the pediatric hematology patient: a prospective comparison of external venous catheters and subcutaneous ports. Am J Pediatr Hematol Oncol 1991;13: 130–136.
17. Wurzel CL, Halom K, Feldman JG, Rubin LG. Infection rates of Broviac-Hickman catheters and implantable venous devices. AJDC 1991;142:536–540.
18. Wiener ES, McGuire P., Stolar CJH, et al. The CCSG prospective study of venous access devices: an analysis of insertions and causes for removal. J Pediatr Surg 1992;27:155–164.
19. Raaf JH. Results from use of 826 vascular access devices in cancer patients. Cancer 1985;55:1312–1321.

20. Sariego J, Bootorabi B, Matsumoto T, Kerstein M. Major long-term complications in 1,422 permanent venous access devices. Am J Surg 1993;165:249–251.
21. May GS, Davis C. Percutaneous catheters and totally implantable access systems. JIN 1988;11:97–103.

3
Insertion Technique for Long-Term Venous Access Catheters: Percutaneous Subclavian Vein Cannulation

H. Richard Alexander

Patient Selection and Preoperative Preparation
Technique of Percutaneous Insertion
Troubleshooting
    Insertion Site
    Guidewire Insertion
    Sheath/Dilator Insertion
    Catheter Insertion
    Tunnel Length and Cuff Placement
Port Insertion
External Jugular Vein Cutdown
Port Removal
References

Patient Selection and Preoperative Preparation

There are no clearly established criteria for deciding which patients would benefit most from long-term indwelling venous catheters. In general, the decision to place a catheter depends on the nature and duration of intravenous therapy, the anticipated need for repeated blood sample analyses, and patient preference. Typical candidates for placement of long-term venous catheters include patients undergoing intensive therapy, such as autologous bone marrow transplantation or aggressive combination chemotherapy, as well as patients needing protracted intravenous therapy. It has been estimated that in the United States more than 500,000 long-term indwelling venous catheters are inserted each year. This represents an enormous expenditure of hospital resources and financial expense with respect to the initial cost of the device, insertion, and routine maintenance. In addition, the placement and presence of a long-term indwelling vascular access device in a patient is not free of risk and therefore the decision to place a catheter for any patient should be considered carefully.

Frequently, patients who are suitable candidates to undergo placement of a long-term catheter are already receiving potentially toxic intravenous therapy. Therefore, the optimal timing of catheter insertion should be planned for the interval in which the patient has recovered from treatment-related blood dyscrasias or other untoward treatment-related effects. The general condition of the patient should be carefully assessed to maximize the safety of the procedure. A prior history of thoracic procedures, active mediastinal disease such as Hodgkin's disease, previous radiation therapy to the chest, or multiple previous bilateral central lines should alert one to the possibility that the venous anatomy of the chest may be abnormal. In these situations preoperative evaluation of venous patency may be useful so that an appropriate insertion site can be selected. Successful imaging of thoracic venous anatomy can be performed with digital subtraction angiography, duplex doppler ultrasound, computed tomography, or magnetic resonance imaging.[2-4] Knowledge of the patient's pulmonary reserve, the presence of malignant pleural effusions, prior pulmonary resection, or extent of metastatic disease to the lung may help in directing on which side a long-term venous catheter may be most safely inserted (Table 3-1). The insertion of a catheter into an area of prior surgery that has involved extensive skin flap dissection, such as mastectomy, or through irradiated skin should be avoided as it may predispose the patient to a subsequent infectious complication.

The past administration of various chemotherapeutic agents may have produced subclinical organ impairment which should be appreciated prior to catheter placement. However, a clinical situation that occurs more frequently is the existence of significant neutropenia or thrombocytopenia secondary to recent administration of chemotherapeutic agents. In general, the insertion of long-term venous access catheters should be considered an elective procedure and therefore

TABLE 3-1
Factor Affecting Which Side May Be Safest for Percutaneous Subclavian Vein Insertion of Long-Term Vascular Access Devices

Clinical Feature	Site of Insertion
Large pleural effusion	Ipsilateral
Prior pulmonary surgery	Ipsilateral
Extensive unilateral parenchymal cancer	Ipsilateral
Mastectomy	Contralateral
Radiation field	Contralateral
Cutaneous metastatic disease	Contralateral

performed when conditions are optimal for any particular patient. Recovery of absolute neutrophil counts greater than 1500/mm³ typically indicates return of host immunocompetence and represents a time when catheter insertion can be performed without concerns that the development of febrile neutropenia or severe line sepsis may precipitate early catheter removal.[5] Patients whose catheters are inserted during periods of neutropenia have a higher incidence of septic episodes than in those without neutropenia.[6] Patients with infection should not undergo catheter placement until appropriate antibiotic treatment has been initiated and clinical evidence of infection has resolved.

Thrombocytopenia is frequently encountered in cancer patients and secondary functional platelet disorders may exacerbate a relatively mild low platelet count. Long-term venous access catheters can be safely inserted in the presence of thrombocytopenia[7] and, in general, platelet transfusion perioperatively to 50,000/mL will minimize the incidence of postoperative hemorrhagic complications. Occasionally, patients with refractory thrombocytopenia who do not respond well to platelet transfusion will need long-term venous catheters. In this setting, venous cutdown on the external jugular, cephalic, or internal jugular vein may be the safest approach.

Malnutrition, other medications, or concurrent illnesses such as human immunodeficiency virus (HIV) infection can produce prolongation of prothrombin or partial thromboplastin time. Although mild abnormalities of one parameter, 1 to 2 seconds, does not necessarily require correction, preoperative administration of fresh frozen plasma or vitamin K may be necessary for more severe abnormalities.

Technique of Percutaneous Insertion

Most venous access devices can be inserted safely in an operating suite on an outpatient basis. The operating room suite provides the optimal sterility and cardiopulmonary monitoring equipment. If the procedure is performed in a standard fashion by someone familiar with the catheter and technique of insertion the entire procedure should take less than 30 minutes. Catheters can be inserted using a local anesthetic with monitored anesthesia sedation. If the procedure can be done expeditiously, the anesthesiologist can use a relatively short-acting sedative. The patient subsequently can recover quickly and be released from the recovery area. Despite any amount of experience with catheter insertion, there are occasional procedures that can be prolonged because of a number of technical difficulties and for this reason an operating suite is preferable for prolonged patient monitoring and the availability of additional instruments if needed. Fluoroscopy should be available to confirm appropriate catheter placement during the procedure. In addition, it is essential to test the catheter lumens for ease of infusion and aspiration. Occasionally, despite what appears on fluroscopy to be a normally placed catheter, there is an inability to aspirate easily. This is frequently resolved by slightly repositioning the catheter 1 or 2 cm.

The preferred technique and most accessible site of insertion is the percutaneous method of Seldinger using the subclavian vein. Percutaneous placement can be performed more quickly and with comparable safety to an open venous cutdown.[8,9] The patient is placed supine with a rolled towel between the scapulae to extend the shoulders. The precordium is prepped in a sterile manner and a local anesthetic is infiltrated intraclavicularly. It is optimal to enter the subclavian vein laterally to maximize the space between the clavicle and the first rib (Figure 3-1). With the patient in the Trendelenburg posi-

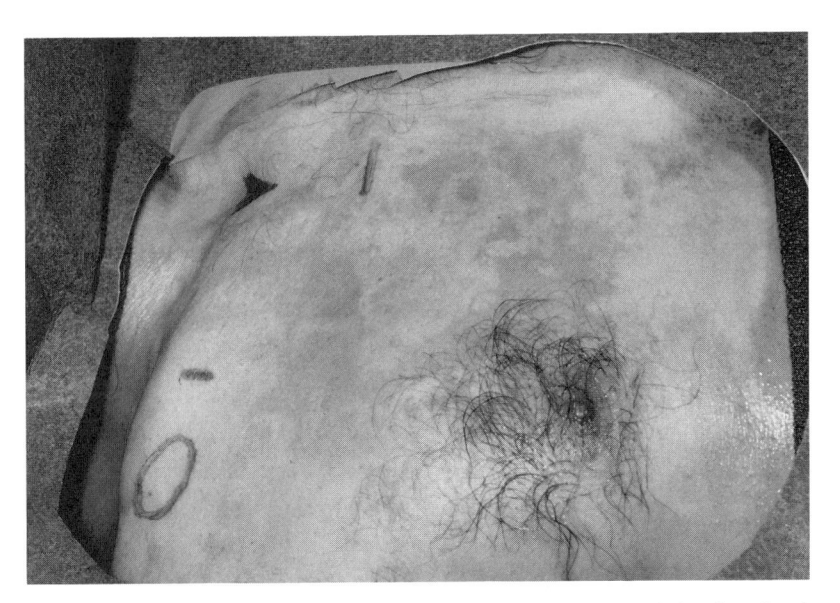

FIGURE 3-1. Photograph of patient illustrating external landmarks for placement of a long-term venous access catheter via the subclavian route. The patient's head is to the left. The sternal notch is marked by an arrow. The angle of Louis and the midportion of the clavicle are marked and the ideal insertion site for the percutaneous subclavian vein cannulation is outlined by the circle. Note the lateral position of the cannulation site to insure that the catheter is not pinched by the scissoring action of the clavicle on the first rib near the costoclavicular ligament.

tion, a needle is advanced into the vein with the bevel up while one gently aspirates on the attached 6-cc syringe. Entry into the vein is confirmed by flow of venous blood into the syringe at which time the needle is rotated 90°, the syringe is disconnected taking care not to allow air to be entrained into the vein through the needle, and a flexible guidewire is advanced through the needle. If pulsatile backflow of blood is observed through the needle the subclavian artery has been cannulated and, after removal of the needle, direct pressure for several minutes should provide adequate hemostasis. If resistance is encountered after the flexible wire has been advanced 2 to 3 cm, the needle is most likely not in the vein. This is illustrated occasionally by noting the wire coiled in the subcutaneous tissue on fluoroscopy as one attempts to advance the wire. In this situation, the needle should be withdrawn with the wire to avoid the possibility of shearing the wire.

After the wire has been successfully advanced, its appropriate position can be confirmed with fluoroscopy. At this point a site on the precordium is selected for the exit site, infiltrated with anesthetic, and the catheter is tunneled through the subcutaneous tissue to the insertion site so that the Dacron cuff is situated subcutaneously approximately 2 cm. above the insertion site (Figures 3-2 to 3-4) The skin adjacent to the wire insertion site is then incised slightly and a peel-away sheath/vessel dilator is gently advanced over the wire. It is very important to ensure that the sheath dilator is threading over the wire

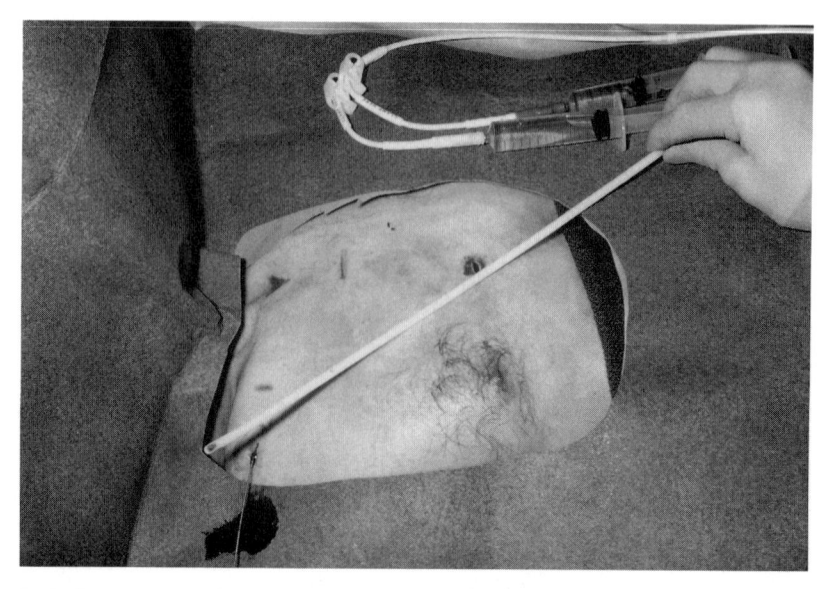

FIGURE 3-2. After cannulation of the subclavian vein and insertion of the J-wire, an exit site on the precordium is selected so that the patient can easily see and care for the catheter. The catheter is tunneled subcutaneously from the exit site to the insertion site as shown. The patient's head is to the left.

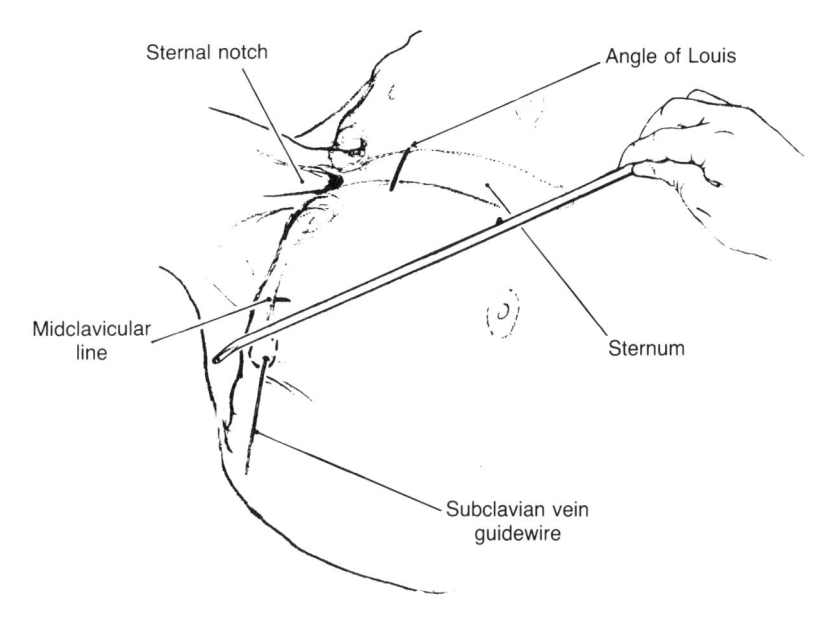

Insertion Technique for Long-Term Venous Access Catheters 43

FIGURE 3-3. Line illustration of the photograph in Figure 3-2 showing the landmarks more clearly.

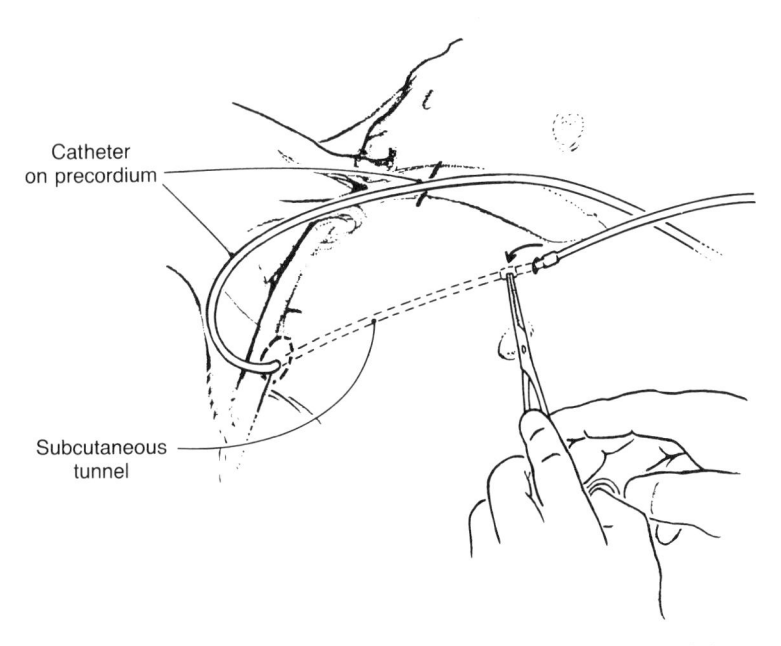

FIGURE 3-4. Illustration showing the preferred final location of the Dacron cuff in the subcutaneous tunnel approximately 2 cm above the exit site.

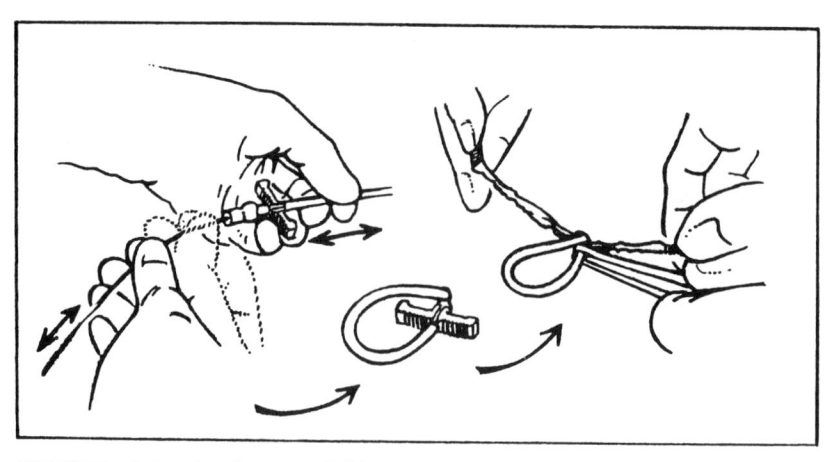

FIGURE 3-5. As the vessel dilator/peelaway sheath complex is advanced into the vein the guidewire should constantly be moved to and fro to ensure that the sheath/dilator is coursing along the path of the wire to minimize the possibility of injury to major mediastinal vascular structures.

by intermittently advancing and withdrawing the wire slightly and checking for resistance (Figure 3-5). It is possible for the sheath dilator to bend the wire and for the surgeon to advance the dilator through the mediastinal vascular structures. This could result in a vascular injury to the mediastinal vascular structures which can result in fatality in these patients.[10] Ideally the catheter tip should lie at the superior vena caval/right atrial junction or just inside the right atrium (Figure 3-6). A higher rate of catheter failure because of occlusive or thrombotic complications has been noted when the catheter tip was high in the superior vena cava or subclavian vein compared to catheters with the tip located in the right atrium.[11] The catheter is cut to its estimated desired length as determined from external bony landmarks. Typically the right superior vena caval/right atrial junction will lie approximately 4 to 6 cm inferior to the angle of Louis (Figure 3-7). By approximating the course of the catheter through the vein on the patient's chest the correct length can be determined. The catheter is then advanced through the peelaway sheath as the sheath is withdrawn (Figures 3-5 through 3-8). The subclavicular incision is then closed in two layers to provide adequate tissue coverage over the catheter, and prior to closing of the exit site, the catheter is sutured in place with either a subcutaneous or a cutaneous anchoring suture.

Troubleshooting

There are several technical features of percutaneous catheter insertion that deserve emphasis. An appreciation of subtle technical aspects will prevent on otherwise straightforward catheter insertion from

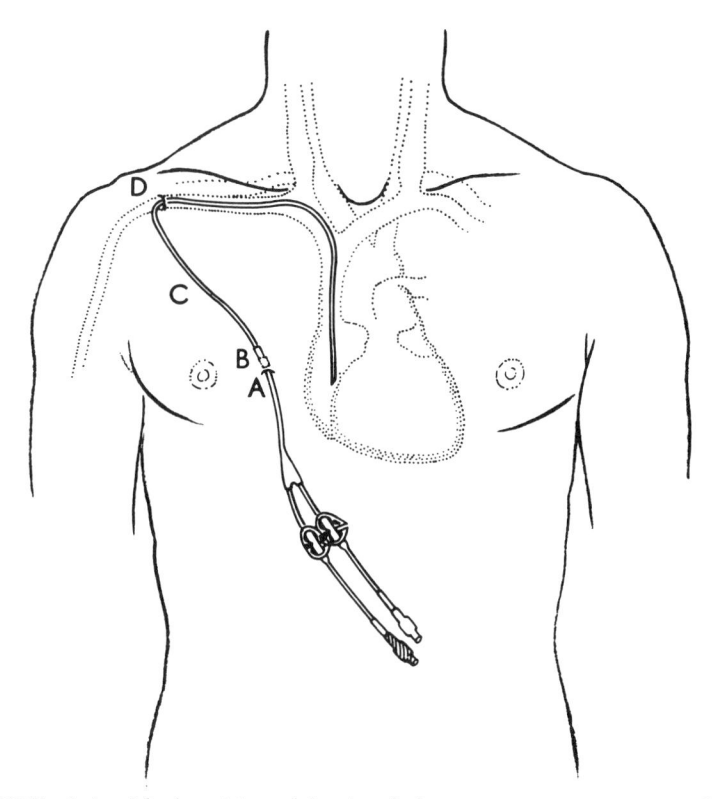

FIGURE 3-6. Ideal position of the tip of a long-term venous access catheter in the area of the proximal vena cava-right atrial junction. The catheter is cut approximately 6 cm below the angle of Louis to approximate its final appropriate intravascular position. The catheter is then inserted into the peelaway sheath and advanced while the peelaway sheath is slowly withdrawn. Occasionally one will meet resistance while attempting to thread the catheter through the peelaway sheath. This may be due to a slight angulation in the peelaway sheath and can often be remedied by withdrawing the peelaway sheath partially while continually advancing the catheter. A, insertion site located so that the patient can inspect and care for catheter; B, Dacron cuff positioned 2 cm above exit site; C, subcutaneous catheter; D, venous insertion site.

consuming the better part of several hours in the operating room. Clearly, each surgeon should develop a standard approach that should minimize the likelihood of technical mishaps.

Insertion Site

The insertion site into the subclavian vein is important. In the infraclavicular area the costoclavicular ligament (Halsted's ligament) holds the first rib and clavicle in fixed close proximity. If the vein is entered and the wire is successfully advanced at this site, the space for the catheter (typically 9.6-French) is very limited and advancing or manipulating the catheter may be very difficult. In addition, there is

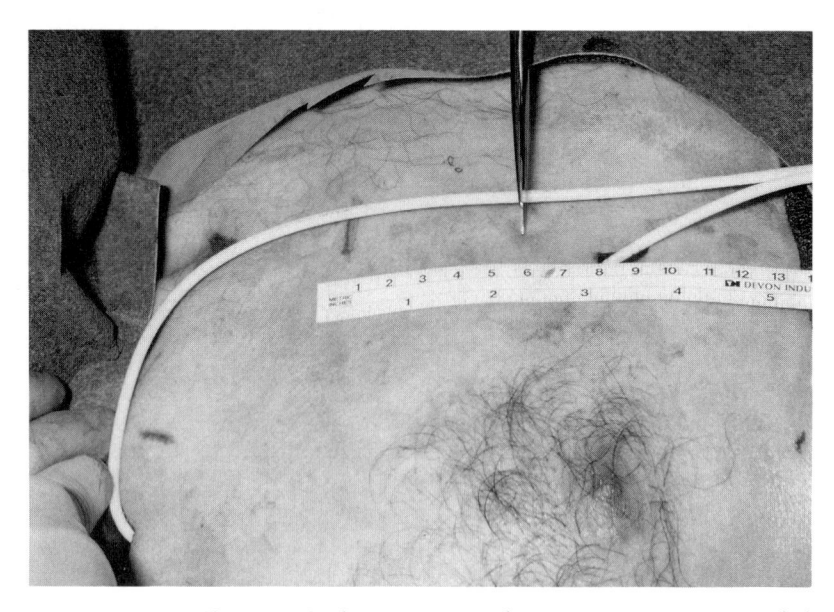

FIGURE 3-7. Photograph demonstrating the approximate course of the long-term venous access catheter on precordium. The catheter is cut approximately 6 cm below the angle of Louis to approximate a final position in the right atrial-superior vena cava junction. The angle of Louis is marked on the precordium. The patient's head is to the left.

the additional risk of catheter pinching or even fracture due to a scissoring effect at this site. To avoid this problem the vein should be entered more laterally (Figure 3-1).

Guidewire Insertion

If the needle used to puncture the subclavian vein is connected to a syringe with a Luer lock mechanism, it may be difficult to disconnect the needle without dislodging it from the vein. Although many insertion kits provide a syringe with a luer lock it may be easier to use a syringe without one so that it can be disconnected easily. The wire should thread easily into the vein. One might *gently* manipulate the wire in an attempt to advance it but it should not be withdrawn forcefully, otherwise a portion could shear off against the needle. In general, once the wire is inserted one does not need to secure it.

Sheath/Dilator Insertion

The sheath/dilator is rigid and can injure the mediastinal vascular structures if great care is not taken. The sheath/dilator has "memory" and can be slightly curved to conform to venous anatomy (Figure 3-9). If the sheath/dilator does not advance easily, fluoroscopy should be

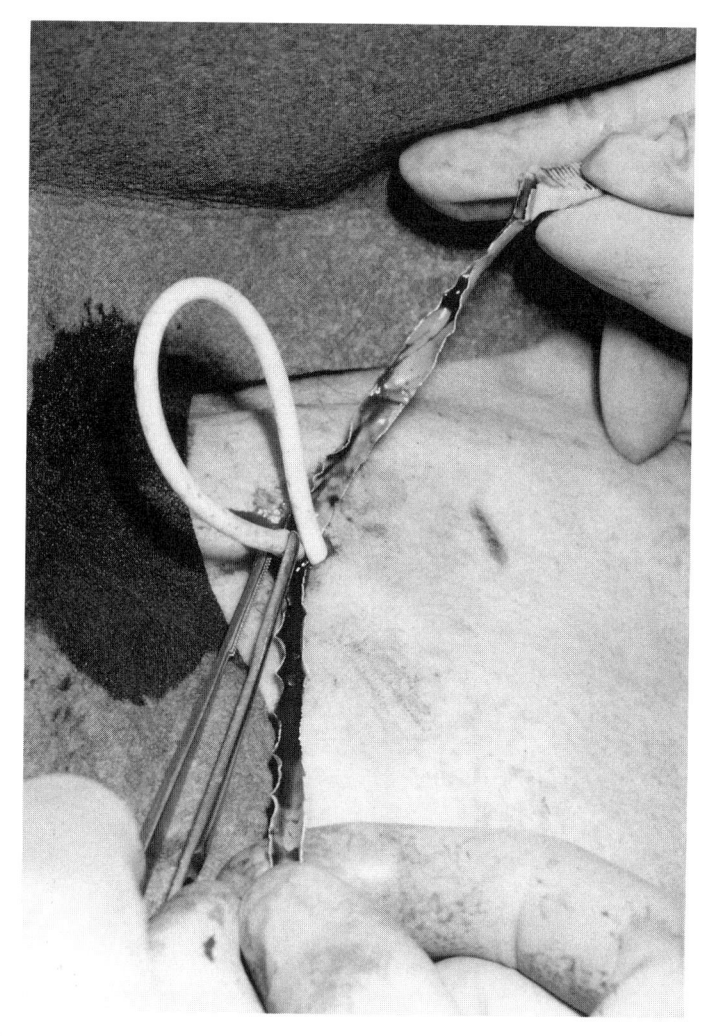

FIGURE 3-8. The Hickman catheter is advanced through the peelaway sheath as the sheath is withdrawn. This technique works well when the catheter cannot be inserted completely into its final position when the peelaway sheath is positioned completely within the vein. Advancement of the catheter through the peelaway sheath can also be facilitated by coating it with sterile mineral oil.

used to check its position. The guidewire should be gently moved back and forth continuously while the sheath/dilator is advanced.

Catheter Insertion

The lumen of the peelaway sheath should be covered with a finger until one is ready to insert the tip of the catheter to minimize blood loss and eliminate the possibility of an air embolism. Occasionally the

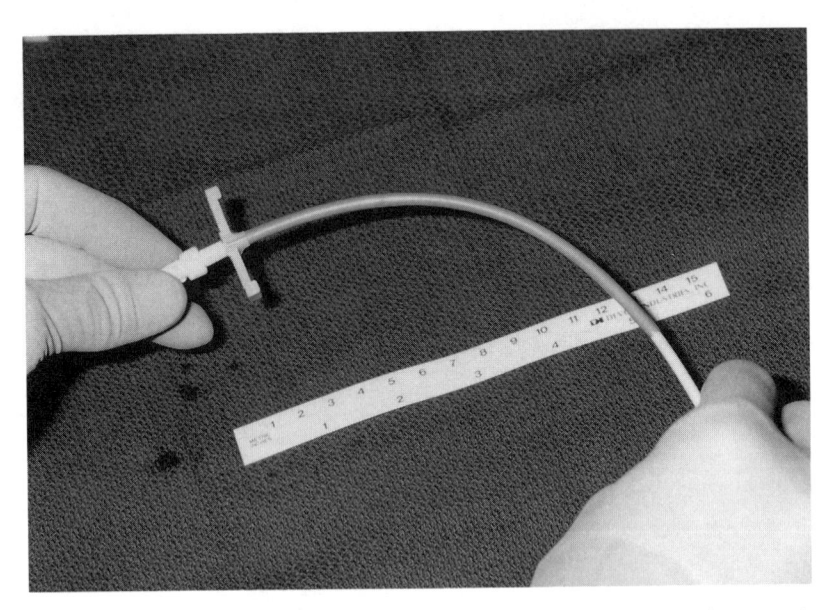

FIGURE 3-9. The sheath/dilator can be curved slightly to conform to the venous anatomy and facilitate advancing it over the guidewire.

catheter will not advance very far into the peelaway sheath. This is most likely secondary to a kink in the sheath or compression as it passes between the first rib and the clavicle. In this case it is helpful to reintroduce the dilator or withdraw the sheath a centimeter or two. Sterile mineral oil can be used also to coat the end of the catheter and facilitate its advancement. Once the catheter is in the intravascular space the peelaway sheath can be partially removed in stages as the catheter is slightly advanced. Fluoroscopy will confirm the proper location of the catheter tip and can be used to reposition a catheter that has been advanced into the contralateral subclavian vein or a neck vein inadvertently. Once the catheter has been inserted into the intravascular space the peelaway sheath should be completely removed if the catheter needs to be manipulated into position. Because the sheath is radiolucent and often stretches as it is pulled out of the vein, it is difficult to know exactly how much remains in the vein. If a small amount of sheath is left in the vein, its relatively stiff character may make manipulation of the catheter into the superior vena cava difficult.

Tunnel Length and Cuff Placement

The exit site should be positioned so that the patient can easily see and care for the catheter. However, care should be taken not to position the exit site so that it is irritated by clothing or causes discomfort for the patient. The incidence of inadvertent catheter dislodgement is higher in adult patients in whom the tunnel is less than 10 cm in

TABLE 3-2
Correlation Between Cuff Position and Patient Age on the Rate of Dislodgment in Pediatric Oncology Patients with Long-Term Venous Access Catheters

Parameter	Percentage of Catheters Dislodged
Cuff position relative to exit site	
≤2 cm	49
>2 cm	28
Patient age (years)	
0–1	18.9
2–3	12
4–7	0.75
>8	0.5

*$P<.009$.
Modified from Wiener ES, McGuire P, Stolar CJH, et al. The CCSG prospective study of venous access devices: an analysis of insertions and causes for removal. J Pediatr Surg 1992;27:155–164.

length and the cuff is placed within 2 cm of the exit site.[12] Weiner has reported similar findings in children with external vascular access devices.[13] In a prospective study from the CCSG of more than 1100 vascular access devices (of which 72% were external catheters), dislodgement was most frequent when the distance from the cuff to the exit site was less than 2 cm and significantly higher than in those children in whom the distance was greater than 2 cm (Table 3-2). Extra precautions to secure the catheter should be taken in very young children because of the higher likelihood of inadvertent removal in this group.

Port Insertion

The principles of insertion for an implantable port are the same as for external devices. The port housing must be placed in a subcutaneous pocket somewhere near the venous insertion site and this is typically located on the precordium. The pocket is fashioned through a 2 to 3-cm incision and extended down to the pectoralis fascia. The port should be anchored to the underlying pectoralis fascia in four quadrants to stabilize the position of the port (Figure 3-10). It should not be placed in very obese patients in whom it would be difficult to palpate and access. The catheter is usually tunneled to the port pocket after insertion and positioning into the vein. However, if the device is preconnected to the port, the port should be placed in the pocket first and the catheter subsequently tunneled up to the insertion site and placed as previously described. The skin over the port should be closed in two layers to maximize tissue coverage over the housing and the housing should be offset so that it does not lie directly beneath the incision.

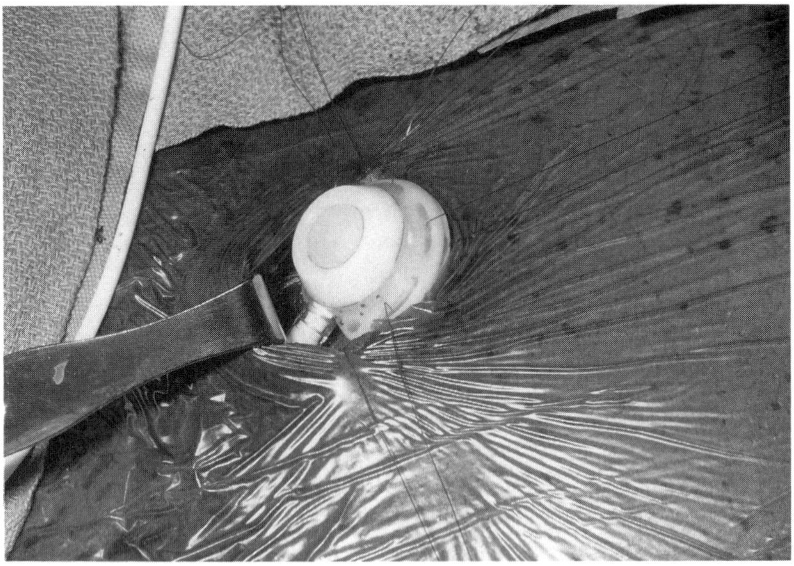

FIGURE 3-10. Port-A-Cath housing with stay sutures placed through the pectoralis fascia and four quadrants being readied for final position within the subcutaneous pocket on the precordium. Four-quadrant fixation is essential to avoid migration or "flipping" of the housing within the subcutaneous pocket.

External Jugular Vein Cutdown

If the subclavian vein is not suitable for catheter insertion then the external jugular or internal jugular vein may be used through a short transverse cervical incision (Figure 3-11). The incision should be made such that it could be extended medially for exposure of the internal jugular vein in the event that the external jugular vein is unsuitable for cannulation.[14] The external jugular vein is just beneath the platysma muscle and can be gently isolated over a hemostat (Figure 3-12). Then 000 silk ties are then placed proximally and distally and the distal tie is ligated (Figure 3-12). When inserting a Hickman style catheter, at this point the catheter should be tunneled from the entrance site on the precordium, over the clavicle, to the venous cutdown site. It is often difficult for the surgeon to assess accurately how much catheter will be needed to position the tip at the right atrial-vena caval junction. In this instance it is prudent to position the Dacron cuff higher in the tunnel prior to placing the catheter in the vein so that in the event that the catheter is slightly too long it can be pulled back and the cuff will remain positioned in the tunnel. The consequence of this maneuver is that, if the catheter is perfectly positioned on the initial try, the cuff will be higher than normal. This really is important onlt at the time of catheter removal, when a small

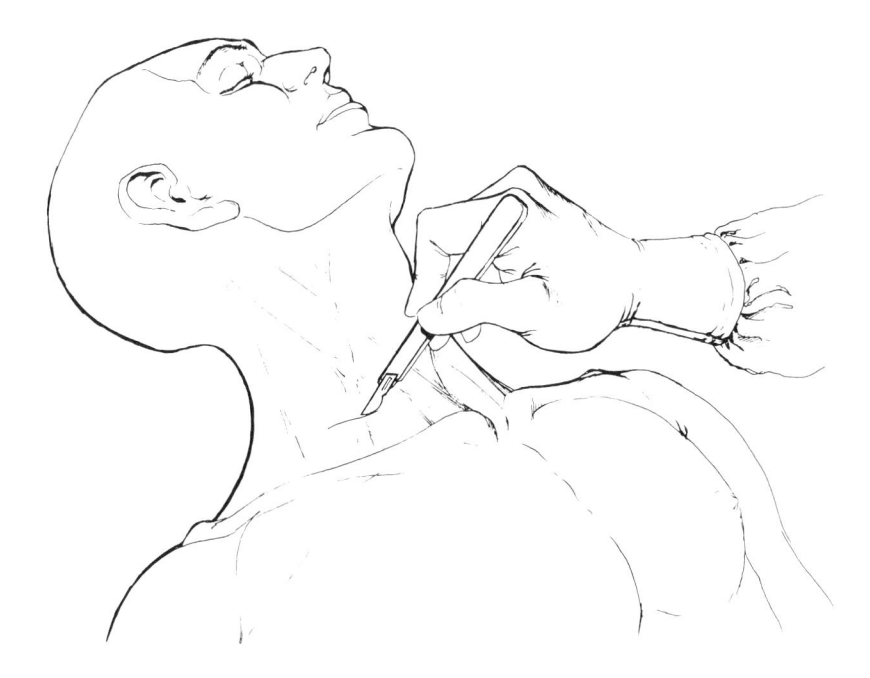

FIGURE 3-11. A short transverse cervical incision is made directly over the external jugular vein low in the neck. In the event that the external jugular vein is not suitable for use, the incision can be extended medially and an internal jugular vein cutdown can be performed.

second counter-incision may be necessary to dissect the cuff from the tunnel.

To successfully, navigate the jugular-subclavian vein junction, it is sometimes helpful to insert a J-wire first which will then stent the vein for the catheter to the superior vena cava. The catheter is secured in the vein by ligating the proximal 000 silk tie. Again the catheter position and function should be checked prior to completion of the procedure.

Port Removal

Removal of an implanted port is often considered a trivial procedure for which a minimal amount of preparation is made. The surgeon does not allocate a realistic period of time for the procedure and may try to do the procedure between outpatients during a busy clinic session. In fact, a small amount of preparation in the way of instruments, lighting, anesthetic, and a standardized approach will keep the procedure from being frustrating for the surgeon and painful for the patient. A standardized technique for removing implanted ports is presented.

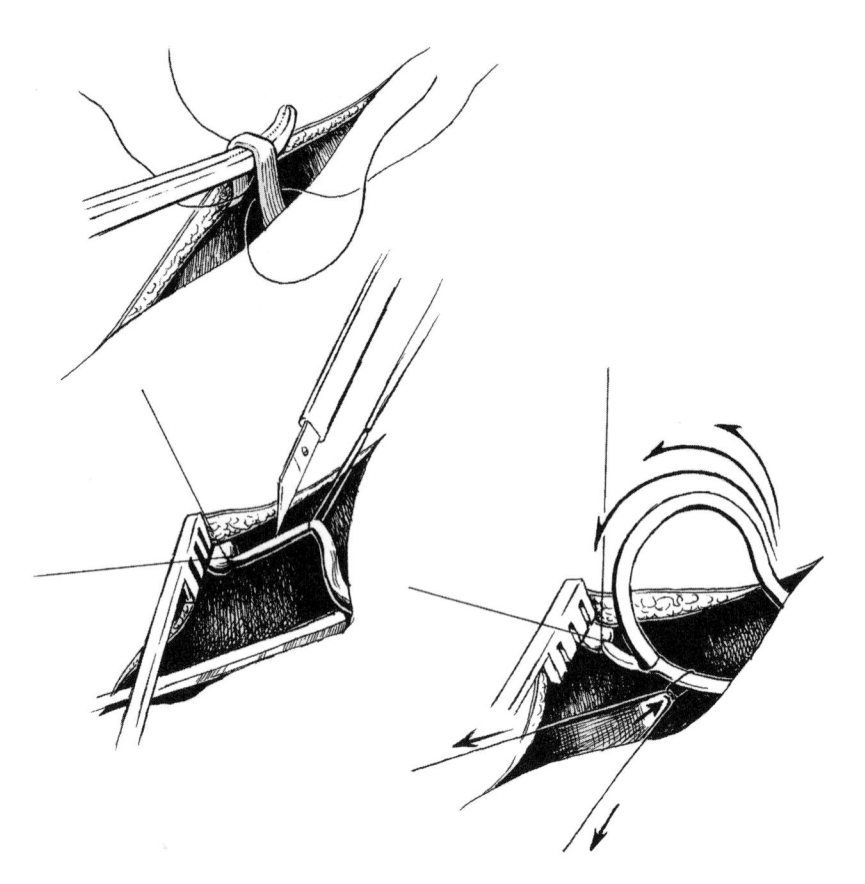

FIGURE 3-12. The external jugular vein is isolated over a hemostat and 000 ties are placed proximally and distally. The catheter is then tunneled from the exit site to the cutdown site. After ligating the distal tie a short transverse venotomy is made and the catheter is advanced into the vein. Occasionally, manipulation of the catheter alone or stenting the vein with a J-wire will help direct the tip into the superior vena cava.

The incision to remove an implanted port should be made through the insertion incision unless the port has migrated somewhat. In this instance the incision is placed over the area where the port housing is connected to the catheter (Figure 3-13). Dissection is carried down until the connection between the port and the catheter is well exposed. This frequently requires a scalpel to incise through the tough pseudocapsule. The housing and catheter can then be grasped with a hemostat (Figure 3-14) and the catheter withdrawn from the vein. This allows one to manipulate the port more freely and facilitates dissection of the pseudocapsule around the housing. The pseudocapsule is frequently very fibrous and must be incised sharply (Figure 3-15). No attempt to remove the surrounding fibrous tissue

Text continues on page 55

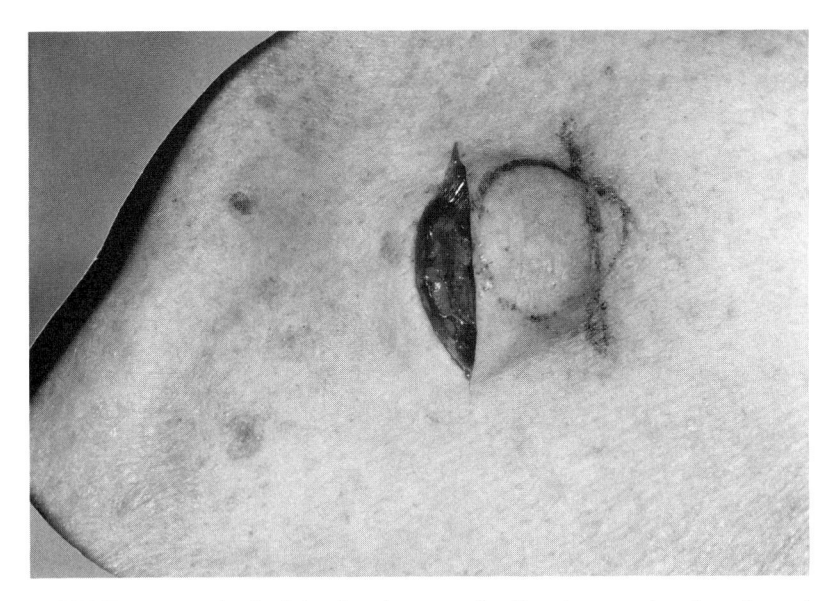

FIGURE 3-13. An incision has been made directly over the site where the port housing is connected to the catheter. During the life of the implantable port the housing has migrated slightly and the original insertion incision has been marked in ink.

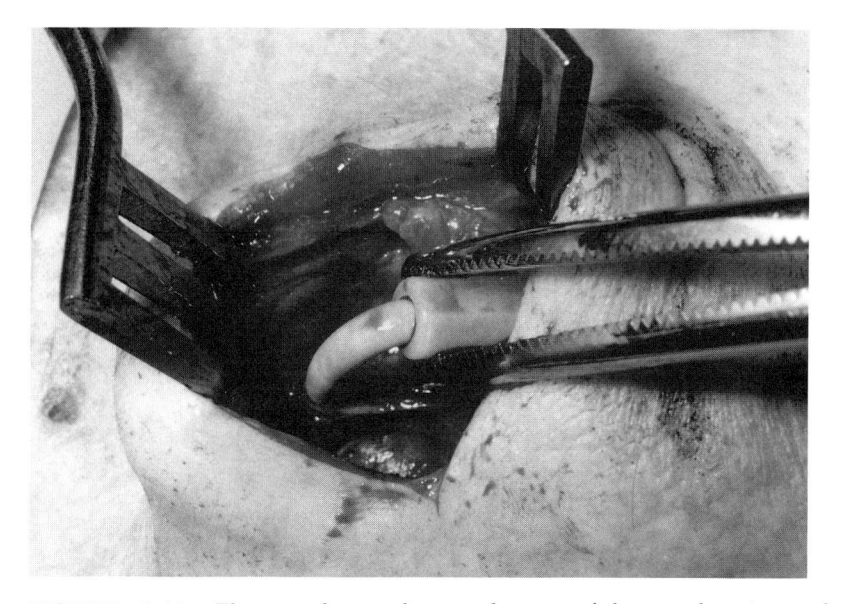

FIGURE 3-14. The pseudocapsule over the area of the port housing and catheter has been incised. The connection between the port and the catheter has been grasped with the hemostat and delivered superficially. The catheter can be removed easily from the vein at this point to facilitate dissection around the pseudocapsule. The port housing has been retracted inferiorly and the pseudocapsule around it is being incised with heavy tissue scissors.

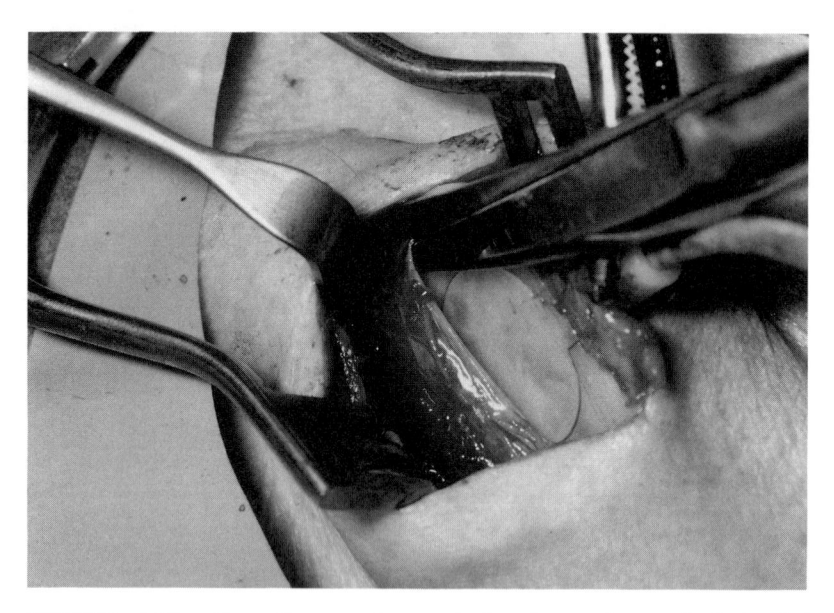

FIGURE 3-15. Once the pseudocapsule has been adequately incised the port will deliver out of the wound easily.

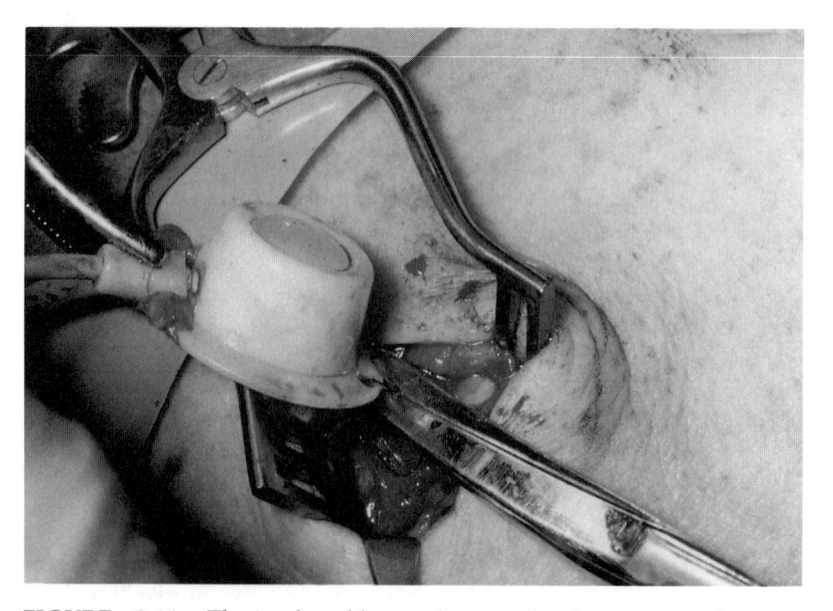

FIGURE 3-16. The implantable port housing has been removed from the pseudocapsule and the remaining stay suture is being divided. Note that no attempt to remove the pseudocapsule has been made. Hemostasis from the subcutaneous pocket and from the venous insertion site is usually spontaneous.

should be made. The anchoring sutures are cut and the port will deliver into the wound easily (Figure 3-16). The wound is irrigated and closed.

References

1. Groeger JS, Lucas AB, Coit D. Venous access in the cancer patient. PPO Updates 1991;5:1–14.
2. Cassidy FP Jr, Zajko AB, Bron KM, Reilly JJ Jr, Peitzman AB, Steed DL. Noninfectious complications of long-term central venous catheters: radiologic evaluation and management. AJR 1987;149:671–675.
3. Chastre J, Cornud F, Bouchama A, Biau F, Benacerraf R, Gilbert C. Thrombosis as a complication of pulmonary-artery catheterization via the internal jugular vein. N Engl J Med 1982;3066:278–281.
4. Falk RL, Smith DF. Thrombosis of upper extremity thoracic inlet veins: diagnosis with duplex Doppler sonography. AJR 1987;149:677–682.
5. Brar KA, Murray DL, Leader I. Central venous catheter infections in pediatric patients in a community hospital. Infection 1988;16:86–90.
6. Hartman GE Shochat SJ. Management of septic complications associated with Silastic catheters in childhood malignancy. Pediatr Infect Dis J 1987;6:1042–1047.
7. Thompson WR, Alexander HR, Martin AJ, Fletcher JR, Ghosh BC. Percutaneous subclavian catheterization for prolonged systemic chemotherapy. J Surg Oncol 1985;29:184–186.
8. Mirro J Jr, Rao BN, Kumar M, et al. A comparison of placement techniques and complications of externalized catheters and implantable port use in children with cancer. J Pediatr Surg 1990;25:120–124.
9. Jansen RFM, Wiggers T, van Geel BN, van Putten WLJ. Assessment of insertion techniques and complication rates of dual lumen central venous catheters in patients with hematological malignancies. World J Surg 1990;14:101–106.
10. Pessa ME, Howard, RJ. Complications of Hickman-Broviac catheters. Surg Gynecol Obstet 1985;161:257–260.
11. Stanislav GV, Fitzgibbons RJ Jr, Bailey RT Jr, Mailliard JA, Johnson S, Feole JB. Reliability of implantable central venous access devices in patients with cancer. Arch Surg 1991;122:1280–1283.
12. Hayward SR, Ledgerwood AM, Lucas CE. The fate of 100 prolonged venous access devices. Am Surg 1990;56:515–519.
13. Wiener ES, McGuire P, Stolar CJH, et al. The CCSG prospective study of venous access devices: an analysis of insertions and causes for removal. J Pediatr Surg 1992;27:155–164.
14. Raaf JH, Heil D. Open insertion of right atrial catheters through the jugular veins. Surg Gynecol Obstet 1993;177:295–298.

4

Long-Term Vascular Access Via Internal Jugular Vein Cutdown

Elizabeth P. Steinhaus

Patient Preparation
Technique of Cut-Down
References

An alternative to the subclavian and external jugular routes for access to the central venous system is the internal jugular vein cutdown. The large number of patients with complex clinical conditions makes this the optimal approach. These patients include those with subclavian veins that are unsuitable because of multiple previous lines, recent line-related infection, or subclavian vein thrombosis. In addition many patients have tissue compromise from previous surgery, metastases, open wounds, or previous radiation on the anterior chest wall, precluding the use of one or the other subclavian vein. Internal jugular vein cutdown allows for superior hemostasis in patients with bleeding diatheses.[1] In addition, the cutdown technique avoids many of the potential complications associated with the blind percutaneous technique including pneumothorax, hemothorax, carotid or subclavian artery puncture, or damage to the thoracic duct.[2]

Patient Preparation

When assessing any patient for vascular access a thorough history and physical examination should be performed. Important historical items include previous catheter insertions and complications associated with them. Multiple previous lines should suggest potential venous scarring or thrombosis. In addition, a history of previous operations or radiation therapy in the vicinity of the vein should be sought. This is important if one is to be aware of potential anatomical deformities of the vein due to radiation injury or the presence of a large mediastinal tumor. The patient's overall health status and coagulation history are also important.

A physical examination can disclose sequelae of venous compromise, such as limb swelling, cyanosis, or the presence of subcutaneous venous collaterals (Figure 4-1).

Radiologic tests aid the assessment as well. Venography can confirm thrombosis of the subclavian vein but is not optimal in patients with renal compromise or previous dye reactions. Doppler ultrasound is safe, noninvasive, and is the optimal study for the internal jugular vein as it can show the caliber of the vein as well as the presence of prograde flow. Once this information has been assembled, an appropriate site can be selected for catheter placement. If both sides are available, the right side is preferable as it is the most direct route, causing fewer problems with catheter malposition and therefore possibly less catheter trauma.[3]

Technique of Cut-Down

The patient is positioned supine with the head slightly elevated. The patient's head is turned at a 45° angle to the contralateral side. This position allows definition of the two heads of the sternocleidomastoid

60 *Vascular Access in the Cancer Patient*

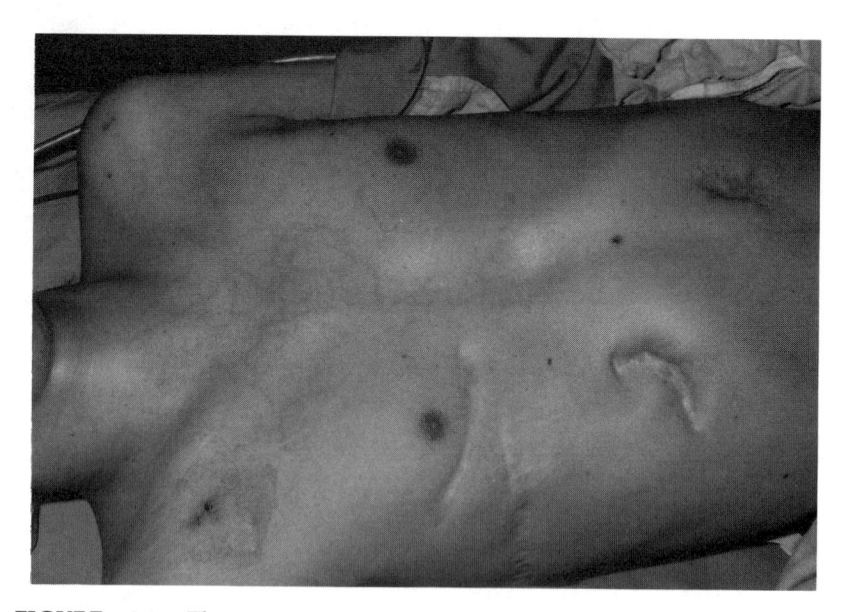

FIGURE 4-1. This patient had undergone placement of multiple previous long-term venous access catheters including a recently infected right subclavian catheter. There was a documented left subclavian thrombosis and the patient had no patent external jugular veins. Note the pattern of subcutaneous veins on the left side of his chest. Doppler ultrasound showed prograde flow without stenosis of his right internal jugular vein.

(SCM) muscle. Landmarks are then defined including the two heads of the SCM muscle, the clavicle, the sternal notch, and the sternal angle (Figure 4-2). If the SCM muscle is not easily appreciated, instruct the patient to turn his head to the ipsilateral side with resistance provided by the assistant or anesthetist. This will sharply demonstrate the two heads so that they can be marked. Draping the ipsilateral nipple into the field helps with longitudinal orientation.

The skin incision is made transversely in the midcervical region approximately 2 to 3 cm above the clavicle.[4] The necessary length of the incision varies but can range from 2 to 5 cm. If one initially attempts an external jugular vein cutdown and is not successful, the incision can be extended anteriorly for internal jugular vein exposure. Electrocautery is used to divide the platysma and the midcervical fascia.[5] The SCM muscle is identified and the clavicular head is retracted laterally. The sternal head may be retracted medially or partially divided if needed for exposure. As the vein can be difficult to identify, palpation of the carotid artery pulse located medially to the vein and observation for the deep blue color of the vein can be used to guide the dissection. Once the vein is identified, care is taken while isolating a segment of vein. Initially a right-angle clamp is placed around the vein allowing an elastic vascular tape to be passed. This tape is then used for gentle retraction of the vein while the remainder of the venous segment is cleared on all sides of the adventitial tissue with sharp dissection. The midportion of the vein generally has no branches which allows safe and easy isolation. Elastic vascular tapes are then placed proximally and distally for control (Figure 4-3).

At this point attention is turned to the chest wall, where a catheter exit site is chosen. Inferior sites are preferred for two reasons. First, the patient can better visualize these sites for catheter care. In addition, accidental dislodgement is associated with shorter cuff-to-exit-site distances[6] and maximizing tunnel length provides the possibility of greater cuff-to-exit-site distance. Local anesthesia is then introduced at the exit site and along the subcutaneous tissue connecting the cutdown and exit sites. Alternatively the systemic analgesia/anesthesia can be deepened for the tunneling maneuver to obviate the need for repetitive needle sticks in a coagulopathic patient. Although we prefer to stay on the ipsilateral chest wall, some suggest a better cosmetic result can be obtained by tunneling to the contralateral chest by way of the sternal notch in order to avoid the catheter running transversely over the edge of the clavicle. A 1-cm incision is made on the chest wall just large enough for insertion of the tunneler. A plastic tunneler supplied with the catheter is used to bluntly connect the two wounds. It is passed subcutaneously over the chest wall and then exits above the clavicle and deep to the platysma between the heads of the SCM muscle. The catheter is then drawn through the tunnel until the cuff is at least 4 cm from the exit wound (Figure 4-4).

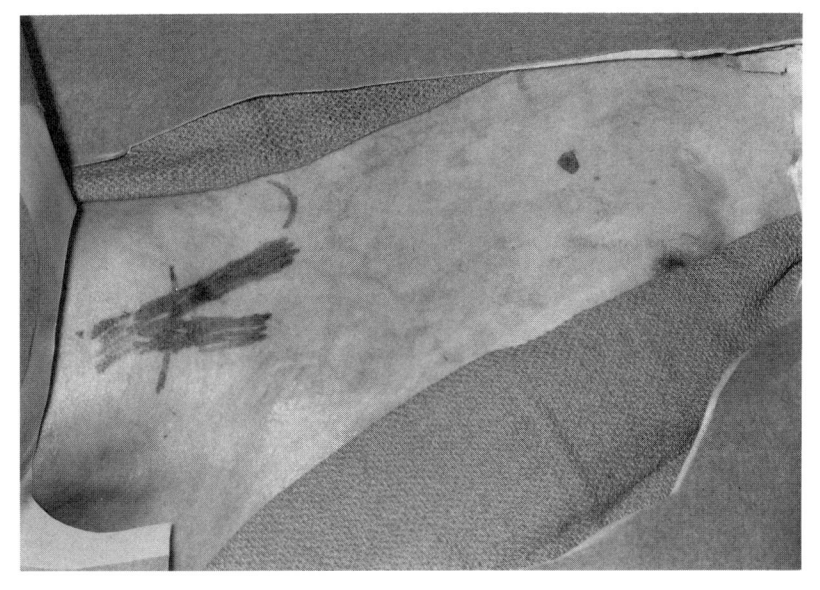

FIGURE 4-2. Landmarks for internal jugular vein cutdown are demonstrated and include the SCM muscle and the sternal notch. The planned incision between the two heads of the SCM is marked. Note that the ipsilateral nipple is draped into the field to help with orientation.

62   Vascular Access in the Cancer Patient

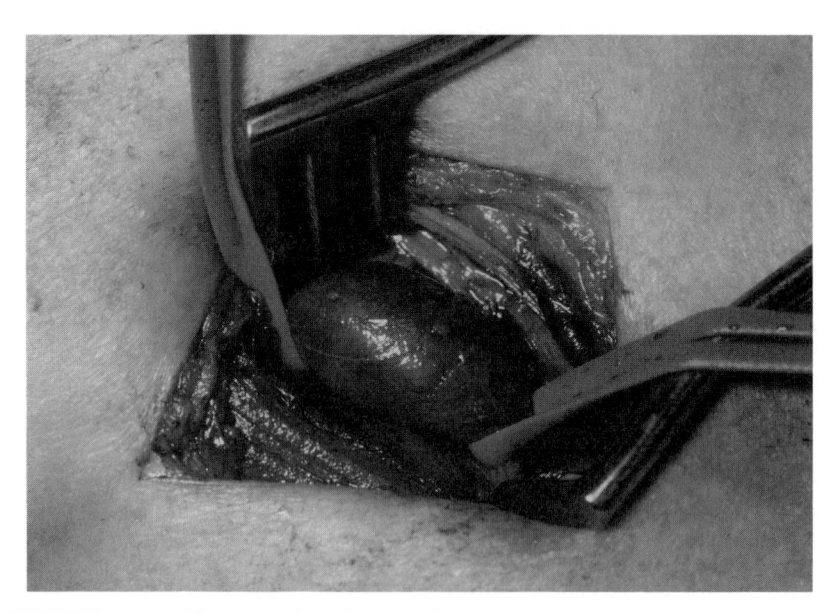

FIGURE 4-3. The sternal and clavicular heads of the SCM muscle can be seen. Vascular tapes around the isolated segment of internal jugular vein deliver it into the wound.

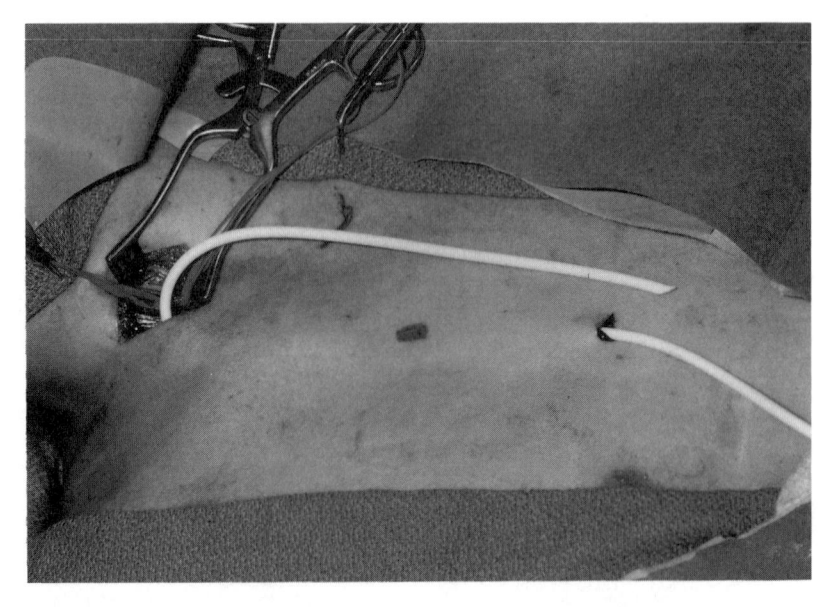

FIGURE 4-4. The catheter is placed subcutaneously through the exit site on the chest wall. The mark midway up the tunnel indicates the location of the cuff at least 4 cm from the exit site. The catheter is then transected at a position approximately 4 cm below the angle of Louis.

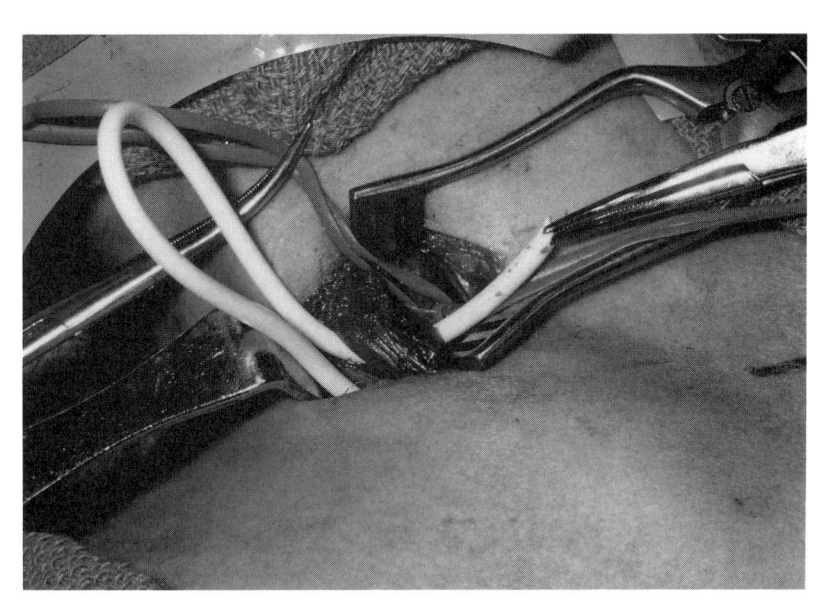

FIGURE 4-5. The catheter is looped beneath the SCM muscle.

The catheter is then transected at a length that will allow placement near the junction of the superior vena cava and the right atrium. The distance to the veno-atrial junction is between 15 and 20 cm from the venous cutdown site. This length is usually estimated by using the length from the venotomy to 4 cm below the sternal angle. The catheter is tunneled under the SCM muscle laterally to help secure its position and maximum soft tissue coverage over the catheter in the area of the cutdown (Figure 4-5).

Attention is then turned back to the vein where the proximal vascular tape is converted to a Pott's occluding tie to secure proximal control. The venotomy tools, which include a venotomy blade and a plastic vein introducer, are then readied (Figure 4-6). The vascular tapes are then retracted bringing the vein up out of the wound and a 0000 or 00000 vascular suture is placed in a pursestring or U-stitch. The suture is placed on the anterior lateral surface of the vein in the center of the wound to allow ease of threading. It is best to allow a generous area (approximately 1 cm) inside the pursestring so that the vein wall will be insinuated between the catheter and the suture. This protects the pursestring from tearing the vein. In the literature some authors have proposed use of an absorbable suture in the vein to avoid trauma to the vein with removal of the catheter.[7] A small venotomy is then made in the center of the pursestring. If necessary Pott's scissors can be used to extend the venotomy. The assistant then uses the vein pick to open the venotomy and the catheter is threaded into the vein. It is important to note that hemostasis is maintained by the vascular tapes above and below. Therefore the lower tape must be

Text continues on page 66

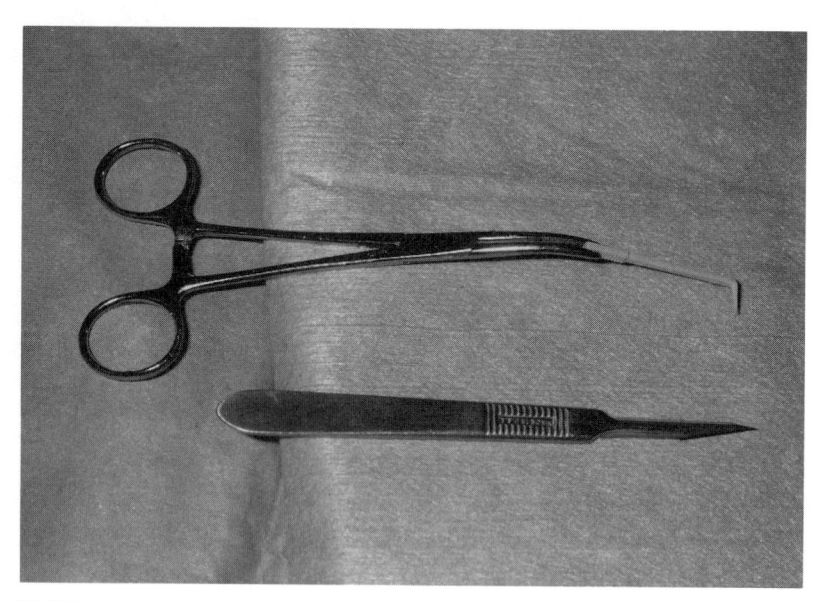

FIGURE 4-6. The instruments for the venotomy are displayed including a venotomy blade and the plastic introducer.

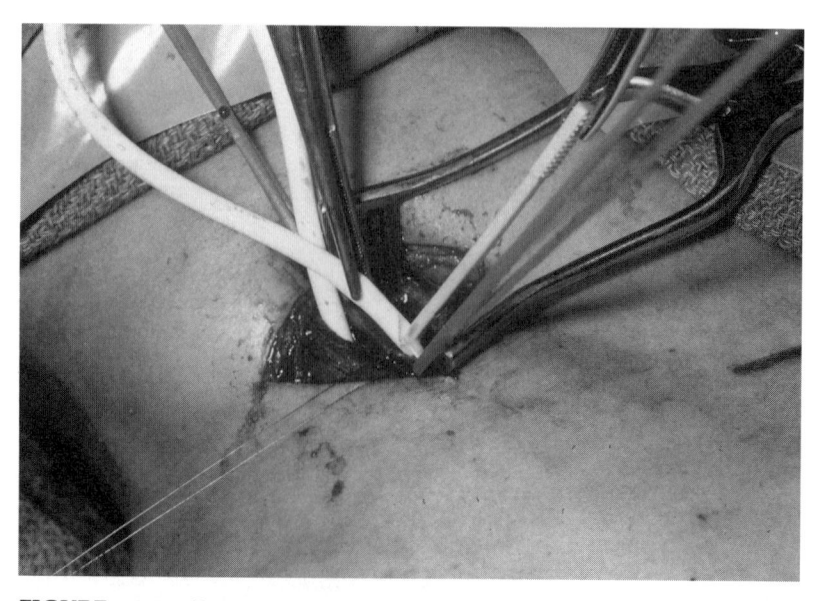

FIGURE 4-7. Forceps are used to introduce the catheter into the vein while the assistant holds the venotomy open.

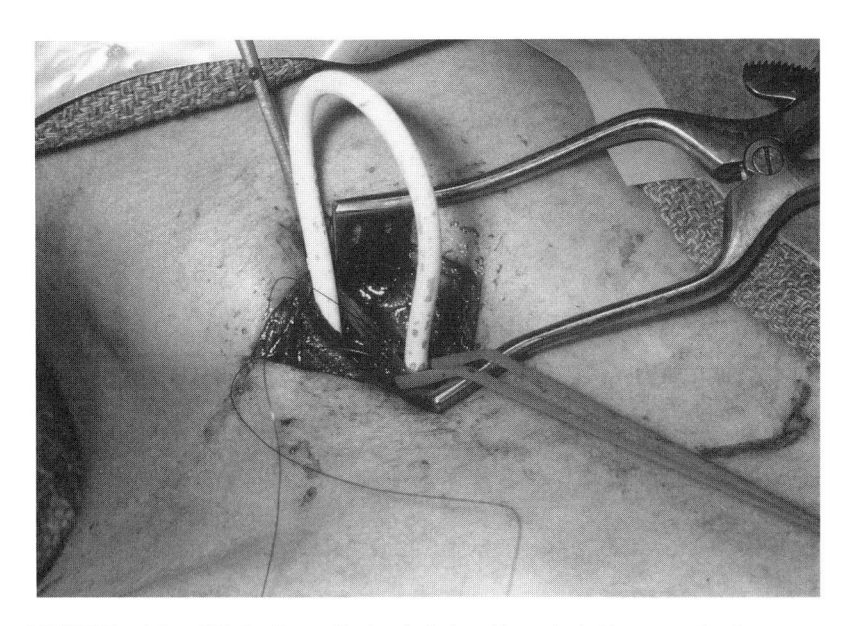

FIGURE 4-8. While the catheter is being threaded, the vascular tapes are held securely but the purse-string is left loose.

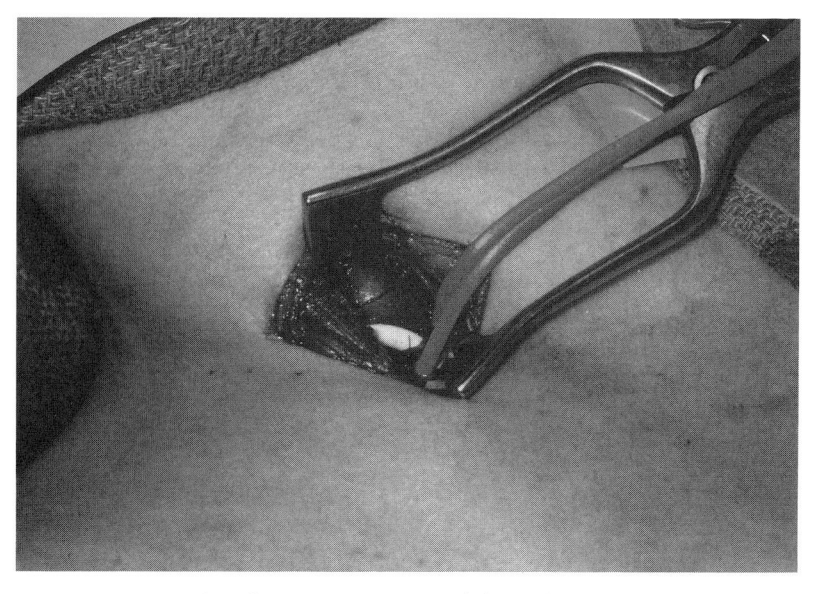

FIGURE 4-9. After the pursestring is tied the catheter is checked for good flow. Before the vascular tapes are removed the venotomy is checked for hemostasis.

quickly loosened and retightened to allow passage of the catheter (Figure 4-7). Tightening the pursestring too early can cause difficulty in advancing the catheter and can tear the vein (Figure 4-8). Only after the catheter has been satisfactorily positioned in the vein should the purse-string be tied (Figure 4-9). Proper placement is then assured with fluoroscopy.

If the catheter has been inadvertently cut too long the intravascular catheter length can be shortened if necessary at this point by 2 to 3 cm quite easily. One possible method is by using local subcutaneous dissection in the neck adjacent to the venotomy site to allow a larger loop of catheter to reside in a subcutaneous pocket external to the vein. The other preferred technique is to pull the cuff inferiorly in the tunnel. This can be done if during the initial placement a generous distance has been left between the cuff and exit site.

Once proper placement is verified the heads of the SCM muscle are closed over the catheter with an interrupted absorbable suture. The platysma is then closed in a similar fashion. At the exit site an absorbable dermal ligature may be placed around the catheter approximately 0.5 to 1 cm up the tunnel. Care must be taken not to compromise the lumens, however, as this may shorten catheter life. The newer catheters come with a suture wing that can be safely secured around the catheter and then sutured to the skin near the exitsite. A chest film is taken postoperatively to document placement and to diagnose any complications.

References

1. Reed WP, Newman KA. An improved technique for the insertion of Hickman catheters in patients with thrombocytopenia and granulocytopenia. Surg Gynecol Obstet 1983;156:355–358.
2. Yakoun M, Joyeux H, Solassol C. Catheterization of the internal jugular vein for total parenteral nutrition. World J Surg 1982;6:369–371.
3. Belcastro S, Susa A, Pavanelli L, Guberti A, Buccoliero C. Thrombosis of the superior vena cava due to a central catheter for total parenteral nutrition. JPEN 1990;14:31–33.
4. Wilson SE, Stabile BE, Williams RA, Owens ML. Current status of vascular access techniques. Surg Clin North Am 1982;62:531–538.
5. Parsa MH, Tabora F. Establishment of intravenous lines for long-term intravenous therapy and monitoring. Surg Clin North Am 1985;65:835–865.
6. Wiener ES, McGuire P, Stolar CJH, Rich RH, Albo VC, Ablin AR, et al. The CCSG prospective study of venous access devices: an analysis of insertions and causes for removal. J Pediatr Surg 1992; 27:155–164.
7. Sagor G, Mitchenere P, Layfield J, Prentice HG, Kirk RM. Prolonged access to the venous system using the Hickman right atrial catheter. Ann R Coll Surg Engl 1983;65:47–49.

5

Difficult Vascular Access: Alternate Sites and Techniques of Insertion

Michael H. Torosian

Simple Solutions
Thoracic Approaches
  Azygos Vein Catheterization
  Superior Vena Cava
  Right Atrium
  Commentary
Inguinal Approaches
  Saphenous Vein Technique
  Femoral Vein Technique
  Inferior Epigastric Approach
  Commentary
Retroperitoneal Approach
  Gonadal Vein Technique
  Translumbar Vein Approach
  Inferior Vena Cava Approach
  Commentary
Angiographic/Surgical Technique
  Commentary
Summary
References

Long-term central venous access has become increasingly common as care is shifted from hospitals to out-patient settings. Parenteral administration of antibiotics, chemotherapy, total parenteral nutrition and other drugs and metabolites has caused a dramatic increase in the number of patients with indwelling central venous catheters. Complications associated with long-term central venous access include sepsis, catheter thrombosis and superior central venous thrombosis.[1-3] Virchow's triad of predisposing factors to venous thrombosis include venous stasis, hypercoagulability and endothelial trauma and are commonly exhibited by patients requiring central venous access. The presence of an intravascular foreign body (ie, catheter) can also precipitate in venous thrombosis.[4,5] The incidence of clinically detectable central venous thrombosis approximates 5% in patients with inwelling central venous catheters.[6,7] Clinically silent central venous thrombi are present in an additional 5–10% of patients as determined by autopsy studies.[8]

In patients with clinically evident central venous thrombosis, venography should be performed to establish the diagnosis.[9,10] After confirmation of the diagnosis, the indwelling central venous catheter is removed and systemic heparinization is begun.[10,11] Embolic complications have been reported in patients with central venous thrombosis and necessitate the use of systemic anticoagulation.[1,10] The anatomic location of the central venous thrombus determines, in part, other available central venous access routes. For instance, unilateral subclavian vein thrombosis permits utilization of the contralateral superior central venous system. However, total or near total superior central venous thrombosis requires use of the inferior venous system or a more innovative approach for insertion of a catheter into the superior central venous system.

The usual routes of access to the central venous system include

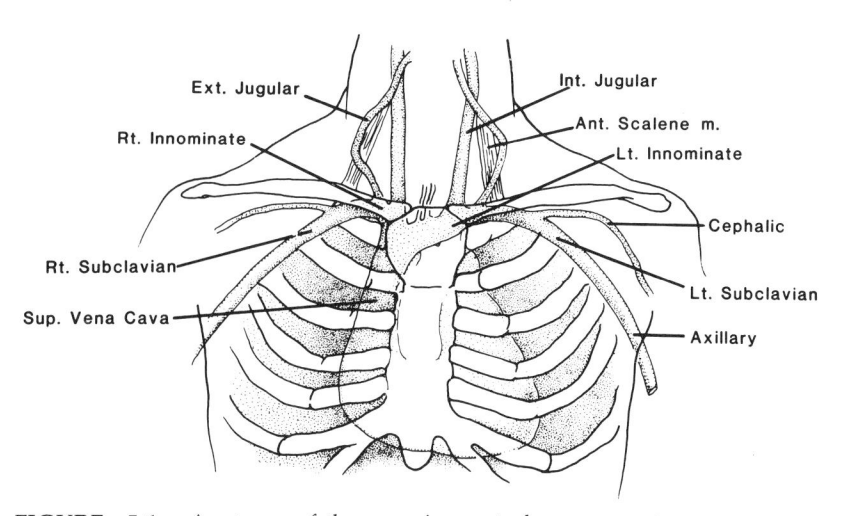

FIGURE 5-1. Anatomy of the superior central venous system.

cutdown techniques to the cephalic, external jugular, and internal jugular veins. Direct percutaneous catheter insertion into the subclavian vein provides a total of eight options for catheter placement in each patient. Following superior central venous thrombosis, head and neck surgery, oropharyngeal fistulae, and upper thoracic or cervical trauma or burns, alternative venous access approaches must be utilized. These alternate approaches for difficult venous access can be grouped into thoracic, inguinal, intraperitoneal, retroperitoneal, and angiographi approaches. Knowledge of alternate routes to obtain venous access is critically important today as the indications for home-based parenteral infusion therapy continue to expand. This chapter discusses the methods of alternate routes of central venous access including advantages, disadvantages, and complications of each technique.

Simple Solutions

If catheter infection or mechanical causes of catheter malfunction necessitate multiple catheter insertions, it is possible to exhaust all of the typical sites of catheter insertion bilaterally. If this situation occurs in the absence of superior central venous thrombosis, several relatively simple solutions exist for reestablishing central venous access. Prior to attempting repeat venous access by the superior central venous route, it is essential to perform venography to establish patency of the central venous system. This diagnostic test will prevent unsuccessful attempts at central venous catheter insertion due to clinically silent episodes of central venous thrombosis. Once venous patency is established, several options for catheterization exist. First, direct puncture of the subclavian vein can be attempted.[12,13] It is frequently possible to reestablish venous access by this technique. Second, additional venous tributaries exist that may be accessed in individuals in whom the cephalic, internal jugular and external jugular veins have been utilized. Such veins include the pectoral vein, thyrocervical vein, and common facial vein.[14-16] Unnamed collateral vessels frequently develop in such patients due to increased collateral venous blood flow. Collateral tributaries that exist close to the subclavian vein occasionally can be accessed by simple cutdown techniques. Finally, when these options fail and it is known that the subclavian vein is patent on the side at which catheter insertion is being attempted, direct cutdown onto the subclavian vein is possible[17] (Figure 5-1). A pursestring suture is placed on the inferior wall of the subclavian vein, a venotomy is made within the pursestring suture, and the catheter tip is advanced through this venotomy and positioned in the superior vena cava. In this way, central venous access can be relatively easily obtained under local anesthesia. Thoracotomy, catheterization of the inferior vena cava, and angiography-assisted catheter insertion can be avoided in this way.

Thoracic Approaches

Thoracotomy with direct catheterization of the superior central venous system or right atrium can be performed in patients who present with difficult angio access problems.[18-20] The first reported case of direct right atrial catheterization for total parenteral nutrition was performed in a patient with superior central venous thrombosis and sepsis caused by a catheter placed in the right femoral vein in proximity to a colostomy.[18] As neither the superior nor inferior central venous systems proved adequate for vascular access in this patient, thoracotomy and direct catheterization of the right atrium was performed. A similar technique can be performed with direct cannulation of the azygos vein.[19] Access to the azygos vein can be achieved either through a retro- or an intrapleural approach.[19,20] The tip of the catheter can then be placed into the root of the superior vena cava (if not thrombosed) or the right atrium.

Azygos Vein Catheterization

Malt and Kempster described direct azygos vein catheterization by a posterolateral thoracotomy incision in the fifth intercostal space.[19] This initial report described an intrapleural approach in which the right upper pulmonary lobe was retracted inferiorly to identify the azygos vein (Figure 5-2). A tributary of the azygos vein is isolated and a right-angle clamp placed beneath the vein to mobilize a small segment from the surrounding soft tissue. Two nonabsorbable sutures are placed around the tributary to be cannulated to achieve proximal and distal vascular control. A Hickman catheter is then tunnelled subcutaneously from an anterior chest wall exit site chosen for ease of patient management after catheter insertion. The catheter is tunnelled through the soft tissue posteriorly and an anterior venotomy is made in the tributary between the nonabsorbable sutures after the distal suture is ligated. The tip of the catheter is then threaded from this site under fluoroscopic guidance through the azygos vein so that its tip will lie in the distal superior vena cava. In this initial report, a 3-cm segment of rib was excised posteriorly for the catheter to exit from the chest cavity. Partial rib resection is not necessary if the catheter is tunnelled above the fifth rib and through the soft tissues of the chest wall.

Angio access through the azygos vein was also described by Pokorny et al in 1984.[20] This report described central venous access in two pediatric patients requiring total parenteral nutrition. In contrast to the intrapleural approach described by Malt and Kempster, a retropleural approach similar to that described for the repair of tracheoesophageal fistulas was used[19,20] (Figure 5-3). A small posterolateral thoracotomy incision was made in the fourth intercostal space with care to remain retropleural. After the catheter is tunnelled through

72 *Vascular Access in the Cancer Patient*

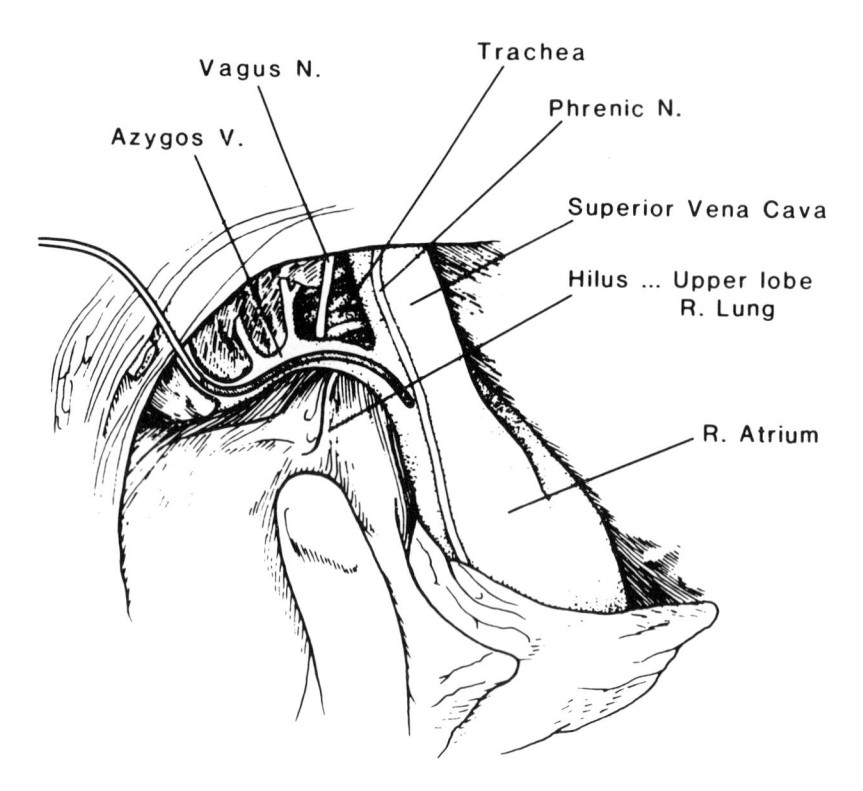

FIGURE 5-2. Intrapleural catheterization of the azygos vein.

the subcutaneous and retropleural space, the azygos vein or one of its tributaries is isolated. Vascular control of the vein is achieved, a venotomy is made, and the tip of the catheter is threaded from this site into the distal superior vena cava. Tube thoracostomy is not required as long as the pleural space has not been violated. This technique provides central venous access through a very proximal central venous tributary without the morbidity associated with intrapleural surgery.

Superior Vena Cava

In patients in whom a thoracotomy has been performed but the azygos vein is found to be thrombosed or unsuitable for cannulation, direct catheterization of the superior vena cava can be performed[17,19] (Figure 5-4). Two nonabsorbable pursestring sutures are placed on the anterolateral wall of the superior vena cava. After tunnelling the central venous catheter from an anterior chest wall exit site, a venotomy is made in the center of the pursestring sutures and the tip of the catheter is threaded from this venotomy site into the distal superior vena cava or right atrium. The catheter is secured to the superior vena

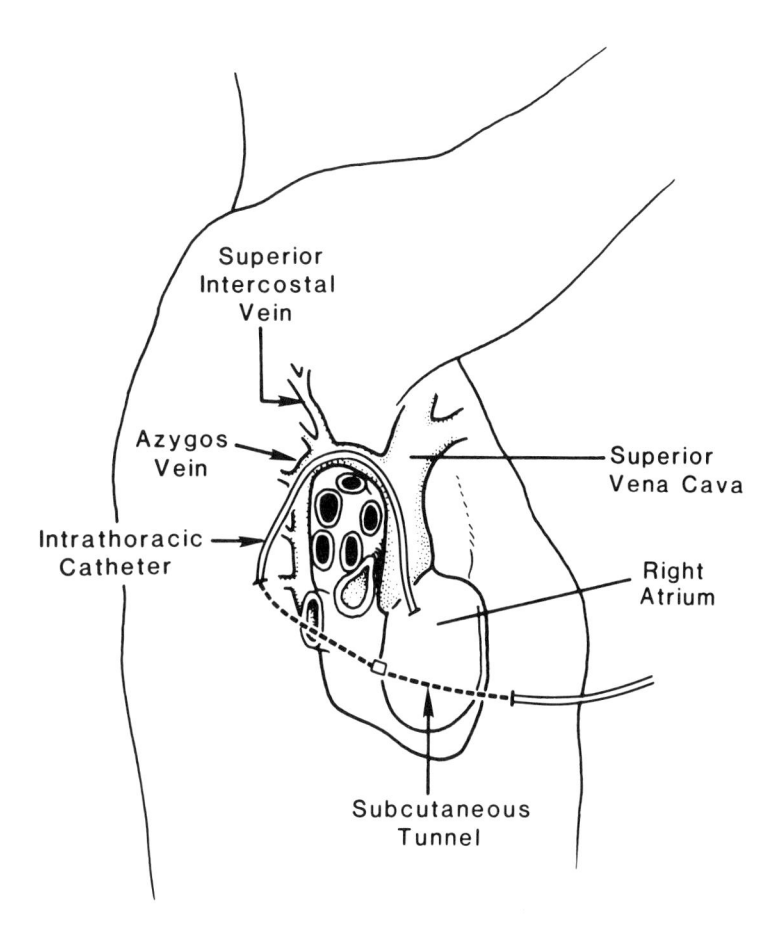

**ANATOMIC RELATIONSHIPS OF
BROVIAC CATHETER PLACEMENT**

FIGURE 5-3. Retropleural approach to the azygos vein.

cava with the pursestring sutures and also to the chest wall with a nonabsorbable suture. This technique has been described but is probably less secure than catheter placement into the azygos vein or directly into the right atrium.

Right Atrium

Direct right atrial catheterization for total parenteral nutrition was first described by Oram-Smith et al in 1978[18] (Figure 5-5). An anterolateral thoracotomy incision was made in the third intercostal space. The pericardium is dissected off the third costal cartilage and the cartilage excised. The pericardium is exposed, incised, and tacked to the subcutaneous tissue with traction sutures. The catheter is tun-

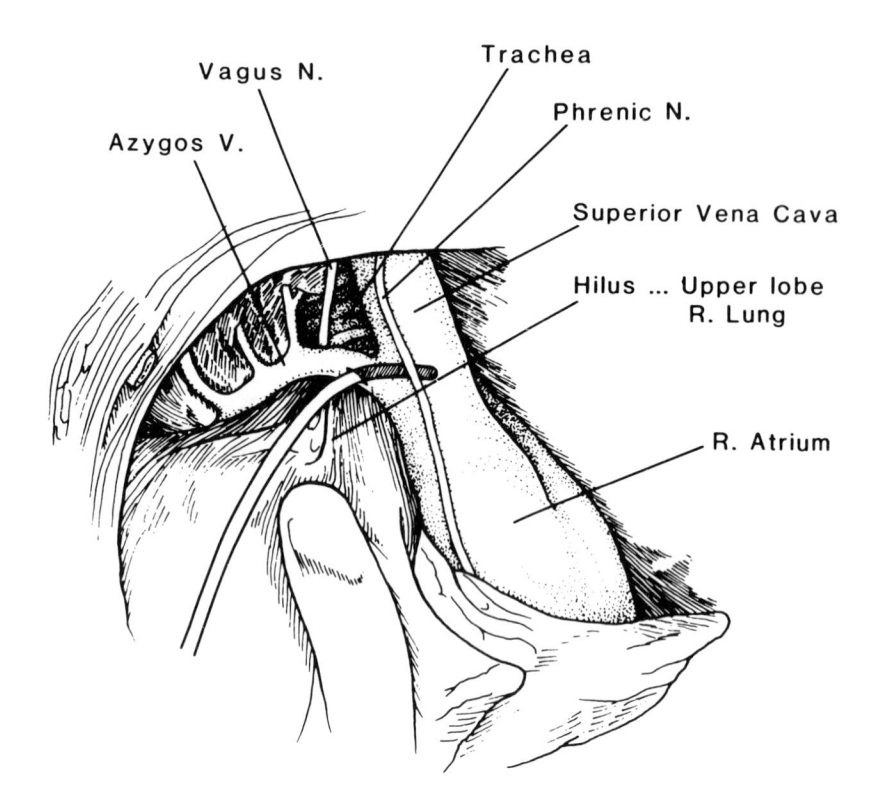

FIGURE 5-4. Direct catheterization of the superior vena cava. Catheter position is secured with two nonabsorbable pursestring sutures.

nelled from an anterior chest wall exit site into the opened pericardium and a pursestring suture is placed around the tip of the atrial appendage. The tip of the atrial appendage is amputated and the distal end of the catheter is placed into the right atrium. Catheter position is secured with several nonabsorbable pursestring sutures. The pericardium and third interspace incision are then closed and the catheter is secured to the skin exit site with a nonabsorbable suture. Although the indications for direct right atrial catheterization are extremely limited, when other options are unavailable, this route can provide an alternative means to establish central venous access.

Commentary

The indications for thoracotomy-based techniques to achieve central venous access are limited. Opening of the pleural cavity is associated with the increased morbidity of pulmonary complications, including atelectasis, pneumonia, and respiratory insufficiency in pulmonary-compromised patients.[21,22] In addition, associated disease processes, such as diabetes, cardiovascular disease, and others in patients requiring long-term central venous access may increase the risk of

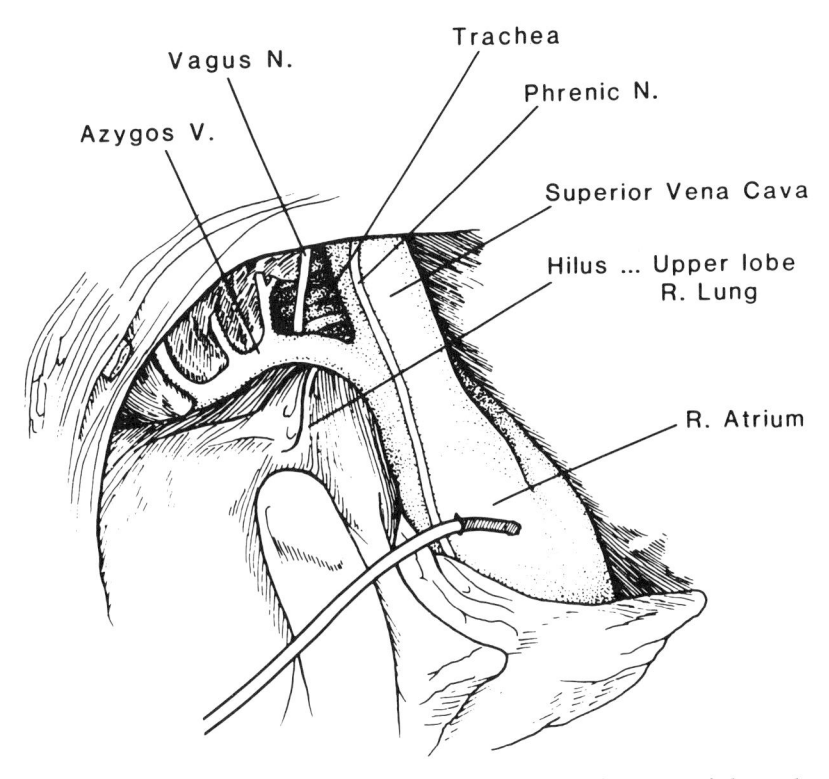

FIGURE 5-5. Catheterization through the amputated stump of the right atrial appendage.

thoracotomy-associated complications.[23] The retropleural approach to the azygos vein or one of its tributaries is attractive because it avoids entry into the pleural space. Perhaps a thoracoscopy-directed technique of catheter insertion will be devised in the future to establish vascular access with minimal morbidity. Nevertheless, each of these options has its indications for use in difficult patients for whom other vascular access sites are unavailable.

Inguinal Approaches

The inguinal approach to the inferior vena cava is the most commonly used technique to obtain central venous access in patients in whom the superior central venous route is not available. Relative contraindications to using the central venous system include venous thrombosis, burns of the head and neck, previous or planned radiation therapy to the neck or mediastinum, extensive cervical or thoracic trauma, oropharyngeal fistulas, and tracheostomy.[24,25] Inguinal access to the inferior vena cava has been popularized by Fondalsrud and others in the pediatric patient population and has been used with increasing frequency in adult patients.[26]

Saphenous Vein Technique

When using the saphenous vein for long-term venous access, there is a possibility of contamination and subsequent infection in the inguinal region. An anterior abdominal wall exit site for the catheter is chosen at least 5 to 10 cm from the inguinal incision.[26-28] An inguinal incision is then made and saphenous vein cutdown performed (Figure 5-6). After the saphenous vein is encircled by two nonabsorbable ties, the distal tie is ligated, an anterior venotomy is performed, and the tip of the catheter is threaded from the saphenous vein into the inferior vena cava. Under fluoroscopic guidance, the tip of the catheter is threaded to the level of the renal veins. The catheter is secured to the saphenous vein with the nonabsorbable ties and the inguinal incision is irrigated and closed in multiple layers. Closure of the soft tissue in multiple layers over the foreign body is essential in the inguinal region to prevent contamination of the catheter by skin organisms in this region.

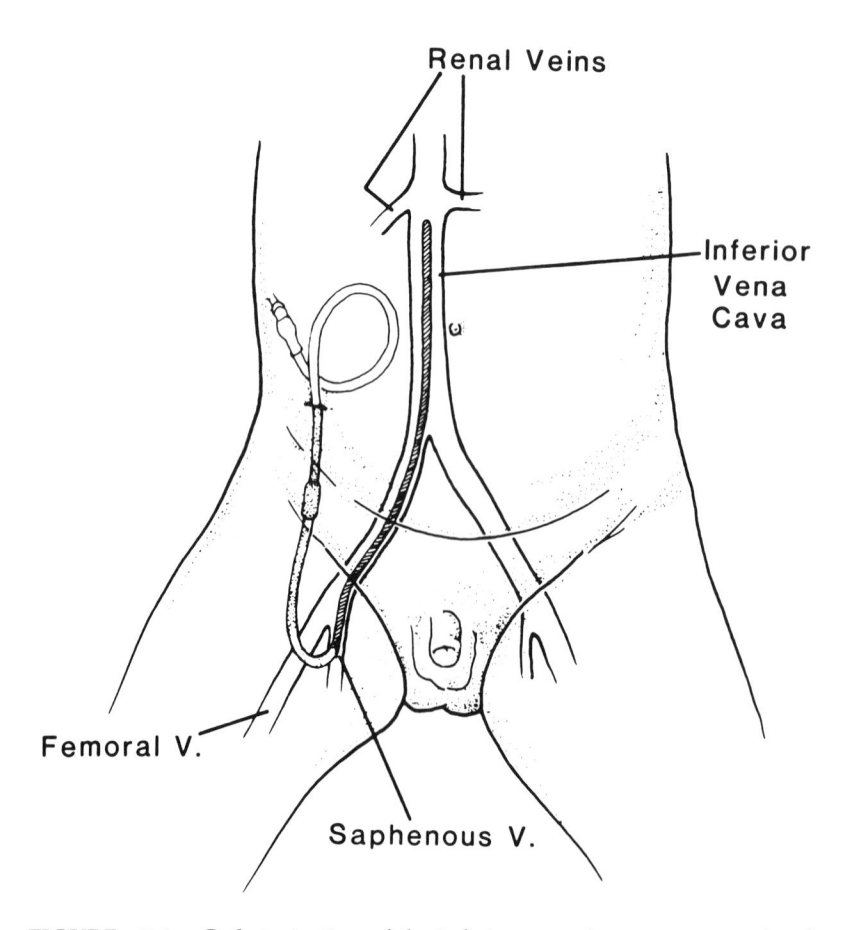

FIGURE 5-6. Catheterization of the inferior central venous system by the saphenous vein.

In a report by Fondalsrud et al, 151 catheters were inserted into the inferior vena cava through the saphenous vein route.[26] In this report, inferior vena cava catheters remained in place through the saphenous vein for a total of 13,288 catheter use days. Infection of the catheter requiring catheter removal occurred in 11 patients. Local signs and symptoms of exit site infection occurred in six patients and evidence of systemic sepsis occurred in five patients. Occlusion of the inferior vena cava developed in four patients—in each of these instances, the catheter had been in place for more than 175 days.[27] No instances of renal vein thrombosis or pulmonary embolism occurred and transient, but not permanent, lower extremity edema was observed. The total incidence of complications in this series was 1 per 225 days of catheter use and complications requiring removal of the catheter occurred in 31 of 151 patients.[26] Thus, ease of catheter insertion in pediatric patients and a comparable incidence of complications to superior central venous access makes this the technique a reasonable option for obtaining long-term central venous access in both pediatric and adult patients.

Femoral Vein Technique

Catheter insertion into the femoral vein can be performed by either a cutdown technique or direct puncture approach.[29] Similar to the saphenous vein approach, an exit site 5 to 10 cm from the inguinal incision is made and the catheter is tunnelled subcutaneously from this site on the lower abdominal wall to the inguinal incision. The femoral vein is exposed and a pursestring suture is placed in the femoral vein (Figure 5-7). A subsequent venotomy is performed and the tip of the catheter is threaded from this site into the inferior vena cava. Alternatively, direct puncture of the femoral vein can be performed with advancement of a guidewire into the inferior vena cava by the Seldinger technique.[29] An introducer with a peelaway sheath is threaded over this guidewire and the tip of the catheter threaded from this site into the inferior vena cava. Several layers of soft tissue are closed over the femoral vein and the catheter is secured to the anterior abdominal wall at the skin exit site. Although large series of these patients have not been reported, direct entry into the femoral vein may increase the incidence of deep venous thrombosis of the iliofemoral system. For that reason, an approach through the saphenous vein or other tributary of the femoral vein are more commonly utilized.

Inferior Epigastric Approach

Isolation of the inferior epigastric vein can be performed on the lower anterior abdominal wall or inguinal region[30] (Figure 5-8). If an inguinal approach is used to isolate the vein, the catheter exit site must be located 5 to 10 cm from the incision. The catheter is threaded from this site into the inferior vena cava by way of the external iliac vein.

78   *Vascular Access in the Cancer Patient*

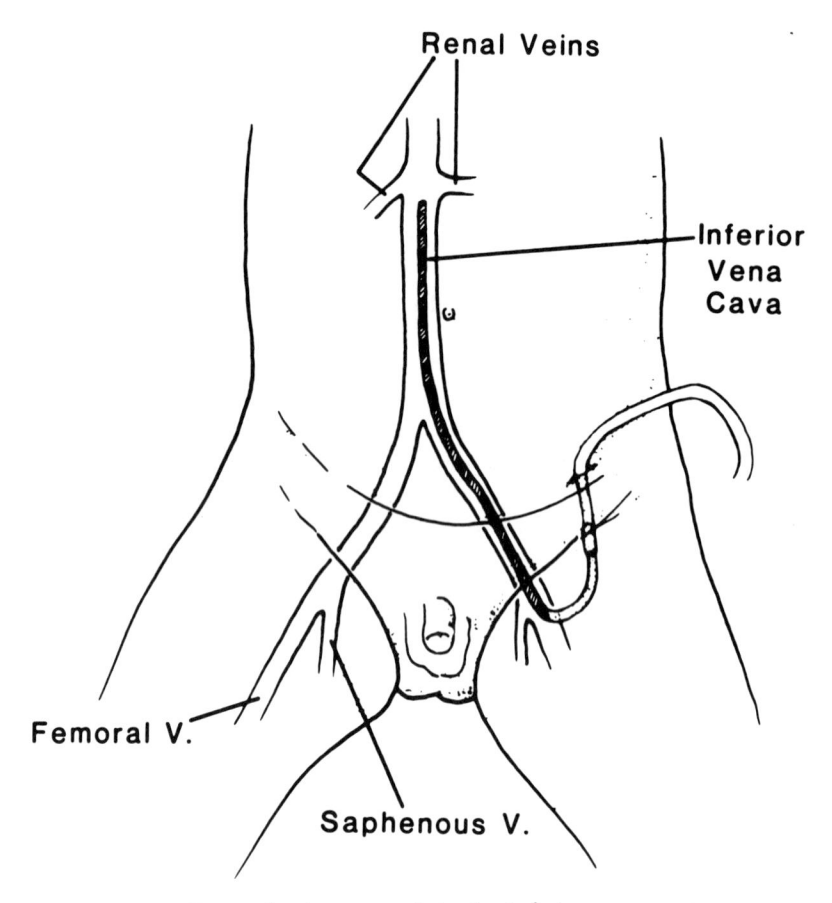

FIGURE 5-7. Femoral vein approach to the inferior vena cava.

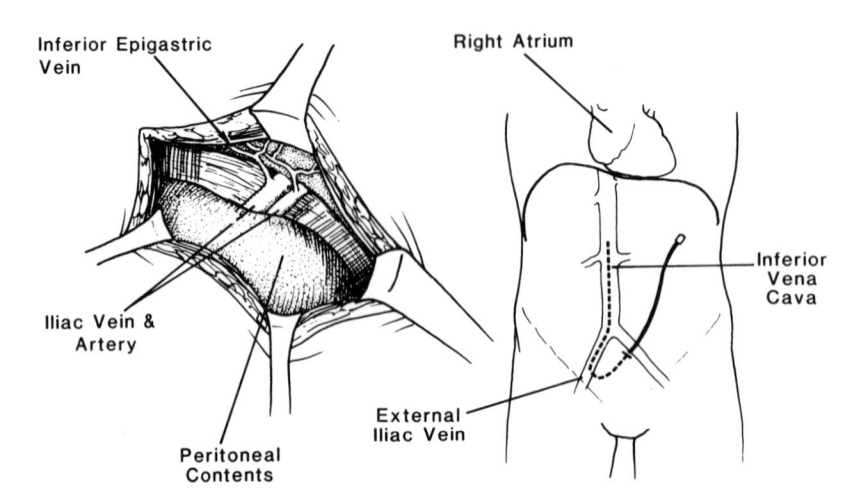

FIGURE 5-8. Catheterization of the inferior vena cava by the inferior epigastric vein.

This is an uncommon technique that is used when other superior and inferior access veins are thrombosed. Second, in contrast to nonambulating infants in whom the saphenous vein approach is commonly used, inferior epigastric vein cannulation can be used in active adults without the need for the catheter to cross the inguinal crease. Thus, there is minimal risk of catheter dislodgement with ambulation. A 5-cm skin incision is made in the line of the skin creases approximately one fingerbreadth above the inguinal ligament in the right or left lower abdominal wall. The catheter is then tunnelled from its exit site 5 to 10 cm away from the skin incision and the catheter brought into the inguinal area. The external oblique fascia is opened and the inferior epigastric vein is isolated just medial to the spermatic cord or round ligament. Cannulation is performed after isolation of the inferior epigastric vein has been obtained between two nonabsorbable ties. An anterior venotomy is made and the tip of the catheter is threaded from this site into the inferior vena cava. Catheter position is confirmed by intraoperative fluoroscopy and the lower abdominal wall incision is closed in several layers. The catheter is then secured to the exit site with a nonabsorbable suture.

Commentary

Inguinal approaches to the inferior vena cava can be accomplished with a low incidence of complications. Williard et al in 1991 reported 31 instances of long-term vascular access through the inferior central venous system.[29] The complication rate was reported at 1 per 254 catheter use days. Major complications included infections (5/31), vascular thrombosis (3/31), isolated catheter thrombosis (3/31), and catheter migration (1/31). The saphenous vein approach is most suited to nonambulating infants whereas the inferior epigastric vein approach can be used in patients with any level of ambulatory status.[26,27,30] Because the course of the catheter remains above the level of the inguinal crease, there is a reduced risk of catheter dislodgement and kinking with the inferior epigastric vein approach. Finally, access by either the saphenous vein or inferior epigastric vein is theoretically preferable to direct cannulation of the femoral vein. The risk of iliofemoral thrombosis, and perhaps pulmonary embolism, exists with endothelial injury to the femoral vein.

Retroperitoneal Approach

The retroperitoneal approach provides another means of access to the inferior central venous system. This route of approach is similar to the inguinal techniques described previously with cannulation of the gonadal and translumbar veins. In patients in whom inferior central venous access is planned, these techniques provide an alternative approach to catheter placement to the inguinal approach. Furthermore, these approaches can be utilized in patients with previous disease- or catheter-induced bilateral iliofemoral thrombosis.

Gonadal Vein Technique

Prior to performing gonadal vein access to the inferior vena cava, inferior vena caval patency should be established by venography. The right gonadal vein is preferable to the left because of its direct takeoff from the inferior vena cava; the left gonadal vein can be utilized but originates from the left renal vein[29,31] (Figure 5-9). After the patient is placed in a supine position with a rolled sheet under the right side, a right flank incision is made. The three muscular layers of the abdominal wall are split in the direction of their fibers and the peritoneum and its contents are swept medially. In the retroperitoneal space anterior to the psoas muscle, the gonadal vein is identified. Care must be taken not to injure the ureter during this procedure. The gonadal vein is cleared of surrounding tissue for a length of 2 cm and two nonabsorbable sutures are placed around the vein to obtain vascular control. An appropriate site is chosen on the anterior abdominal wall for the exit site of the catheter and the catheter is tunnelled from this site to the gonadal vein where an anterior venotomy is made for catheter

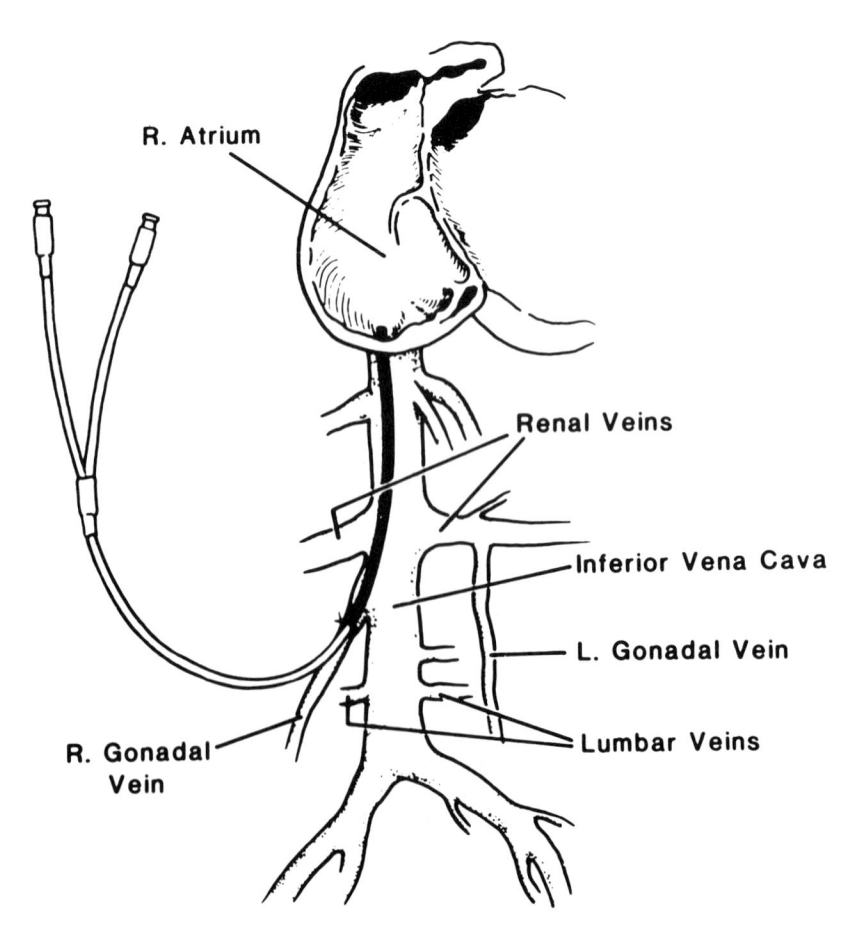

FIGURE 5-9. Gonadal vein catheterization into the inferior vena cava.

entry. The catheter is advanced from this site into the inferior vena cava and ligated to the vessel with the nonabsorbable sutures. The catheter tip is advanced to the junction between the inferior vena cava and the right atrium as determined by intraoperative fluoroscopy. The right flank incision is closed in multiple layers after allowing enough catheter in the retroperitoneal space to allow for traction during ambulation and normal activity after surgery.

Translumbar Vein Approach

An alternative to the gonadal vein approach to the retroperitoneal inferior vena cava is the lumbar vein technique.[32] The patient is positioned with the ipsilateral flank elevated by a roll. A flank incision is made extending anteriorly from the 12th rib, the abdominal wall muscles are split, and the retroperitoneal space is entered. The plane between the peritoneum and the psoas and quadratus lumborum muscles is developed and an appropriate lumbar vein is identified. The lumbar vein is dissected from its surrounding soft tissues and vascular control is obtained with nonabsorbable ligatures (Figure 5-10). After the catheter is tunnelled from its exit site on the anterior

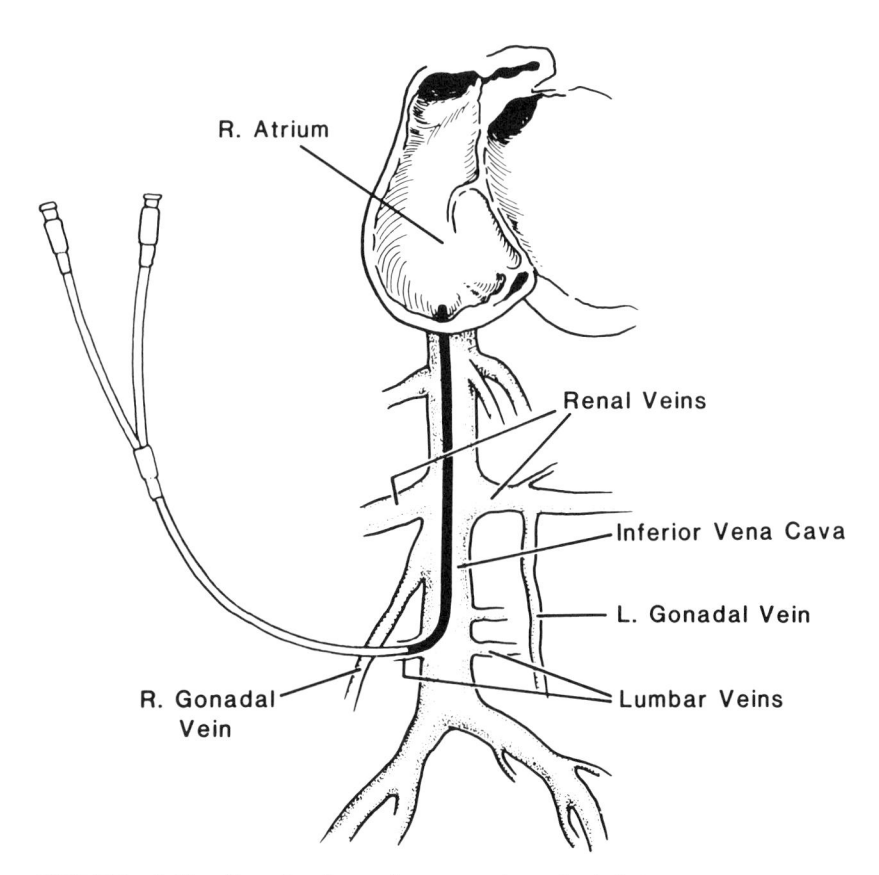

FIGURE 5-10. Translumbar vein approach to the inferior vena cava.

abdominal wall to the retroperitoneal space, venotomy is performed and the tip of the catheter is threaded from this site into the inferior vena cava near its junction with the right atrium. The catheter is secured to the lumbar vein with nonabsorbable ties and the catheter is secured to the abdominal wall at the skin exit site.

Inferior Vena Cava Approach

When the retroperitoneal venous access approach is attempted and neither the gonadal vein nor a lumbar vein can be identified that will accommodate the catheter, direct inferior vena cava cannulation can be performed.[31,33] The inferior vena cava is identified and a pursestring suture is placed at the planned site of catheter entry (Figure 5-11). The catheter is tunnelled from its exit site on the abdominal wall to the retroperitoneal space and inserted into the inferior vena cava at the site of the pursestring suture. This suture is used to secure the catheter to the inferior vena cava. The catheter is advanced to an appropriate level in the inferior vena cava, the incision is closed, and the catheter is secured externally at its skin exit site.

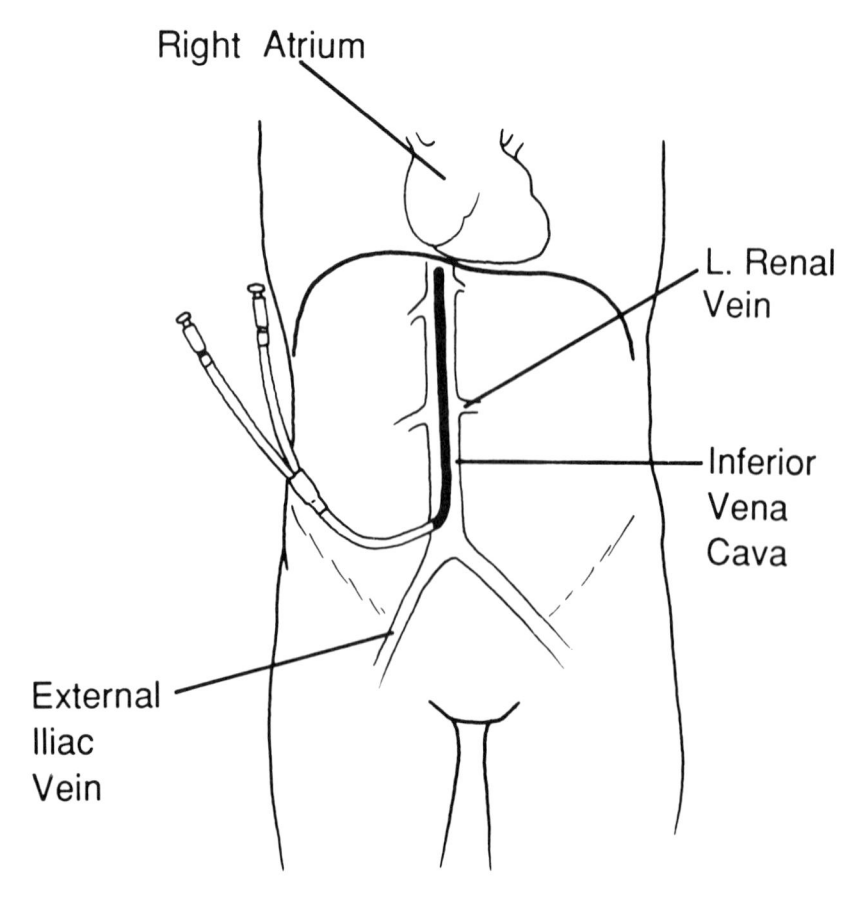

FIGURE 5-11. Direct catheterization of the inferior vena cava.

Commentary

Retroperitoneal vascular access through the gonadal, lumbar, and inferior vena caval approach has several advantages. First, this technique can be used in patients with superior central venous thrombosis or in patients with upper thoracic burns, trauma, or sites of infection in whom superior central venous access cannot be performed. Second, this approach to the inferior central venous system can be performed even in patients with iliofemoral venous thrombosis. Collateral veins including the gonadal vein and lumbar veins are usually dilated in these patients and have excellent blood flow. Third, because of the short distance that the catheter resides within the inferior vena cava, it is suggested that the incidence of inferior vena caval thrombosis may be reduced compared to inguinal access techniques. This theoretical advantage to the retroperitoneal approach has not been confirmed because of the small series of patients reported with gonadal or translumbar catheters.

Angiographic/Surgical Technique

A combined angiographic/surgical technique has been devised to insert an indwelling catheter through a thrombosed superior central venous system.[34] This approach can be performed under local anes-

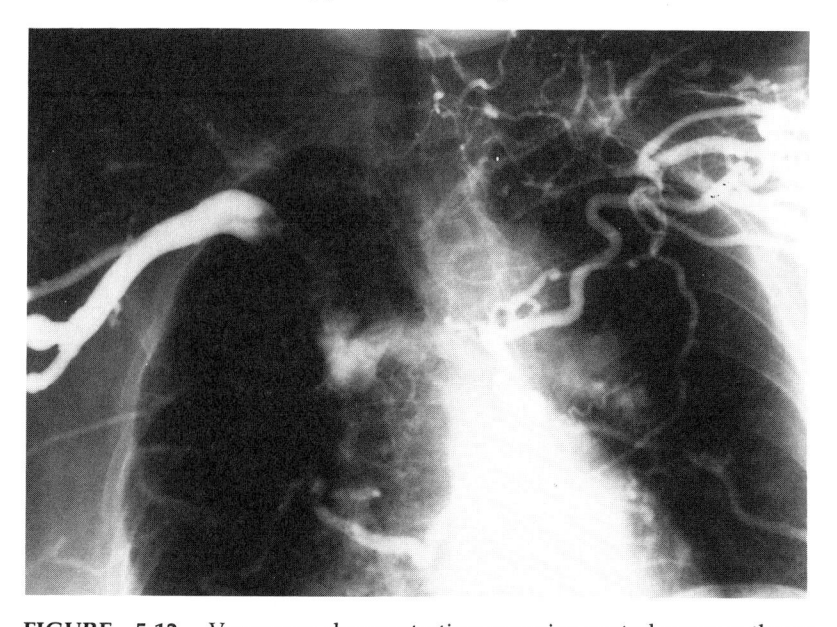

FIGURE 5-12. Venogram demonstrating superior central venous thrombosis with extensive development of collateral vessels. Reprinted with permission from Torosian MH, Meranze S, Mullen JL, McLean G. Central venous access with occlusive superior central venous thrombosis. Ann Surg 1986;203:30–33.

thesia with minimal morbidity and requires both angiographic and surgical expertise. Torosian et al reported three patients in whom catheters had been placed by this technique through a totally occluded superior central venous system-including bilateral subclavian, innominate, and superior vena caval thrombosis[34] (Figure 5-12). The first step involves superior central venous and collateral venography to identify a collateral vein that will be the target for surgical cutdown and insertion of the catheter. The spot on the skin beneath which this collateral vein is located is marked with a lead marker during venography. A guidewire is then introduced by retrograde basilic or femoral vein approach through the occluded superior vena cava into the previously identified collateral vein. In the three instances in which this procedure has been reported, the vein utilized for catheter insertion was the recanalized internal jugular vein, recanalized axillary vein, and an enlarged, collateral eleventh intercostal vein. Once the guidewire has been advanced to the appropriate collateral or recan-

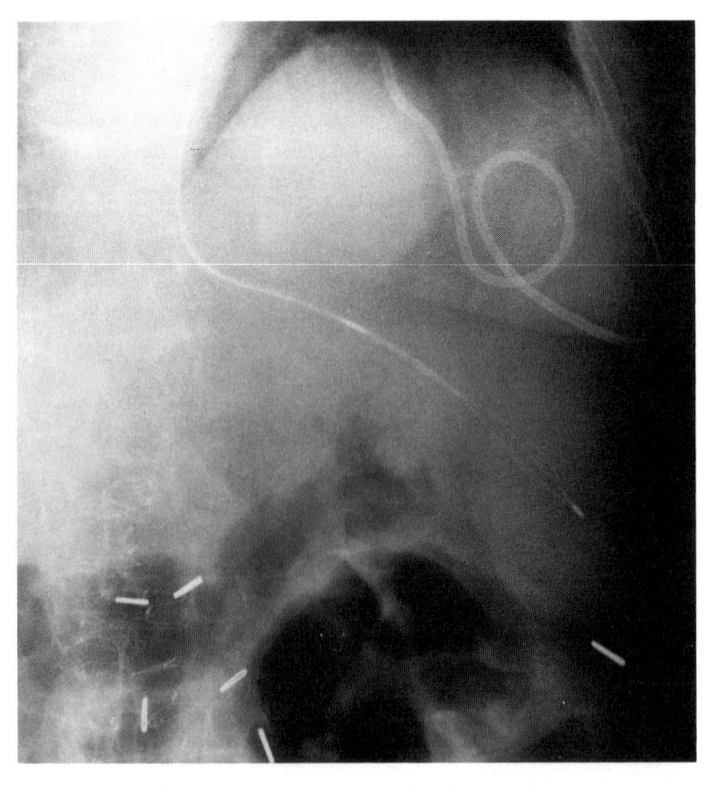

FIGURE 5-13. A Dormia basket catheter has been advanced over a guidewire from the basilic vein and through the thrombosed central venous system to a patent left 11th intercostal vein. 14.Postoperative chest x-ray demonstrating the course of the Hickman catheter from the left eleventh intercostal vein to the enlarged hemiazygos vein.

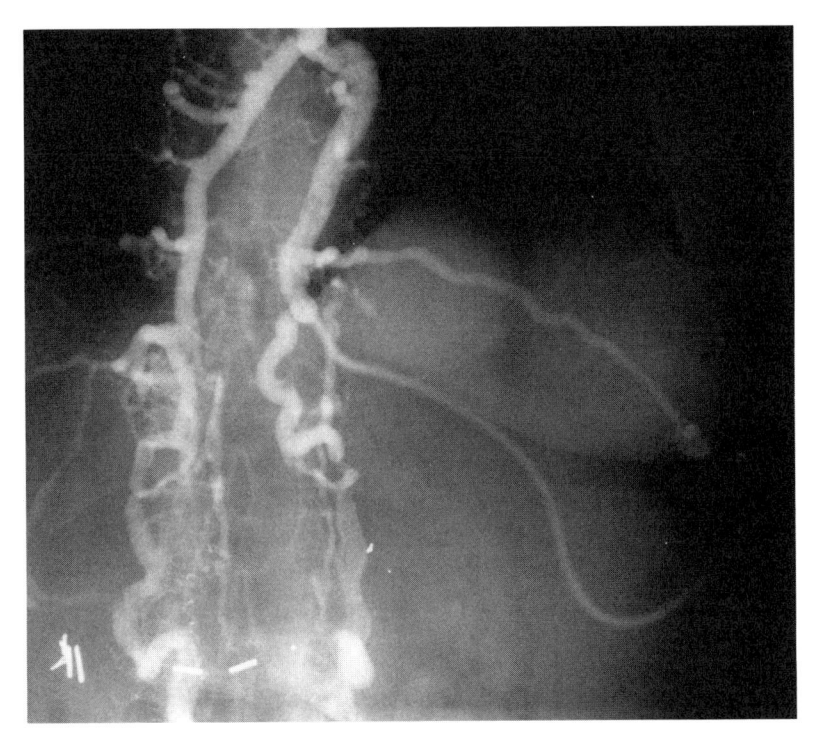

FIGURE 5-14. Postoperative chest x-ray film demonstrating the course of the Hickman catheter from the leflt eleventh intercostal vein to the enlarged hemiazygos vein.

alized vein, the patient is taken to the operating room. The patient is placed in an appropriate position and, under local anesthesia, cutdown is performed at the point previously marked with the lead marker. Dissection is performed to identify the vein containing the guidewire and proximal and distal vascular control obtained with nonabsorbable ties. An appropriate exit site is then chosen on the chest wall and the catheter tunnelled from this site to the incision. The catheter is measured and cut at an appropriate length so that it will lie in the distal superior vena cava or right atrium. A dormia basket catheter is then introduced over the guidewire at the basilic or femoral region and the wire is removed (Figure 5-13). The tip of the Hickman catheter is then grasped by the basket and the basket catheter is slowly withdrawn at the basilic or femoral vein. This is performed under fluoroscopic guidance and, when the tip of the catheter reaches the junction between the superior vena cava and the right atrium, the basket is opened to release the Hickman catheter tip (Figure 5-14). The angiographic catheter is then removed from the femoral vein and the surgical incision closed in several layers. The three catheters placed by this technique and reported in the literature have functioned for over 6, 27, and 38 months, respectively.

Commentary

The combined angiographic/surgical technique requires significant planning and expertise by both angiographic and surgical teams. The advantage to this technique is that it can be performed in a patient with superior central venous thrombosis under local anesthesia. This procedure avoids thoracotomy with its associated morbidity in a patient in whom long-term central venous access is required and catheterization by inferior vena caval approaches is unavailable or contraindicated. No episodes of pulmonary embolism have been observed with this approach.

Summary

Long-term central venous access is commonly used today for parenteral infusion therapy. As this practice becomes more prevalent, increasing episodes of central venous thrombosis will be observed. Numerous alternative routes for obtaining central venous access exist including thoracic, inguinal, retroperitoneal, and combined angiographic/surgical techniques. Innovative techniques will undoubtedly continue to be developed to solve the complex problems presented by patients with prolonged requirements for central venous access.

References

1. Singh AK, Dykvizan DL, Vargas LL. Acute superior vena cava obstruction with intravenous thrombosis: a complication of central venous catheterization. Cardiovasc Dis 1979;6:308.
2. Dillon JD, Schaffner W, VanWay CW, Meng HC. Septicemia and total parenteral nutrition: Distinguishing catheter-related from other septic episodes. JAMA 1973;223:1341.
3. Forlaw L, Torosian MH. Central venous catheter care. In Clinical nutrition. Vol 2: Parenteral nutrition. Philadelphia: WB Saunders, 1985.
4. Hoshal VL Jr, Ause RG, Hoskins PA. Fibrin sleeve formation on indwelling subclavian central venous catheters. Arch Surg 1971;102:253.
5. Peters WR, Bush WH, McIntyre RD, Hill LD. The development of fibrin sheath on indwelling venous catheters. Surg Gynecol Obstet 1973;137:43.
6. Grant JP. Handbook of total parenteral nutrition. Philadelphia: WB Saunders, 1980.
7. Padberg FT, Ruggiero J, Blackburn GL, et al. Central venous catheterization for parenteral nutrition. Ann Surg 1981;193:264.
8. Ryan JA Jr, Abel RM, Abbott WM, et al. Catheter complications in total parenteral nutrition: A prospective study of 200 consecutive patients. N Engl J Med 1974;290:757.

9. Allen JR. The incidence of nosocomial infection in patients receiving total parenteral nutrition. In: Advances in parenteral nutrition. Lancaster, England: MTP Press, 1978.
10. McLean-Ross AH, Griffith DM, Anderson JR, Grieve DC. Thromboembolic complications with silicone elastomer subclavian catheters. JPEN 1982;6:61.
11. Brismar B, Hardstedt C, Jacobson S, Kager L, Malmborg A. Reduction of catheter-associated thrombosis in parenteral nutrition by intravenous heparin therapy. Arch Surg 1982;117:1196.
12. Jesseph JM, Conces DJ Jr, Augustyn GT. Patient positioning for subclavian vein catheterization. Arch Surg 1987;122:1207–1209.
13. Kirkemo A, Johnston MR. Percutaneous subclavian vein placement of the Hickman catheter. Surgery 1982;91:349–350.
14. Kaminski MV Jr. Hyperalimentation: a guide for clinicians. New York: Marcel Dekker, Inc.
15. Kosloske AM. and Klein MD. Techniques of central venous access for long term parenteral nutrition in infants. Surg Gynecol Obstet 154: 395–399. 1982.
16. Zumbro GL, Mullin MJ, Nelson TG. Central venous catheter placement utilizing common facial vein. Am J Surg 1973;125:654–656.
17. Torosian MH. Long-term vascular access. In: Rothkopf MM, Askanazi J (eds): Intensive homecare. Baltimore: Williams & Wilkins, 1992.
18. Oram-Smith JC, Mullen JL, Harken AH, Fitts WT. Direct right atrial catheterization for total parenteral nutrition. Surgery 1978;83:274–276.
19. Malt RA, Kempster M. Direct azygos vein and superior vena cava cannulation for parenteral nutrition. JPEN 1983;7:580–581.
20. Pokorny WJ, McGill CW, Harberg FJ. Use of azygous vein for central catheter insertion. Surgery 1985;97:362.
21. Bria WF, Kanarek DJ, Kazemi H. Prediction of postoperative pulmonary function following thoracic operations. J Thorac Cardiovasc Surg 1983;86:186.
22. Shah DM, Powers SR. Prevention of pulmonary complications in high risk patients. Surg Clin North Am 1980;60:1359.
23. Harmon E, Likington GA. Pulmonary risk factors in surgery. Med Clin North Am 1979;63:1289.
24. Mitchell A, Atkins S, Royle GT. Reduced caheter sepsis and prolonged catheter life using a tunnelled silicone rubber catheter for total parenteral nutrition. Br J Surg 1982;69:420–422.
25. Press OW, Ramsey PG, Larson EB, Fefer A, Hickman RO. Hickman catheter infections in patients with malignancies. Medicine 1984;63:189–200.
26. Fondalsrud EW, Berquist W, Burke M, Ament ME. Long-term hyperalimentation in children through saphenous central venous catheterization. Am J Surg 1982;143:209–211.
27. Fondalsrud EW, Ament ME, Berquist WE, Burke M. Occlusion of

the vena cava in infants receiving central venous hyperalimentation. Surg Gynecol Obstet 1982;154:189–192.
28. Curtas S, Bonaventura M, Meguid MM. Cannulation of inferior vena cava for long-term central venous access. Surg Gynecol Obstet 1989;168:120–124.
29. Williard W, Coit D, Lucas A, Groeger JS. Long-term vascular access via the inferior vena cava. J Surg Oncol 1991;46:162–166.
30. Maher JW. A technique for the positioning of permanent central venous catheters in patients with thrombosis of the superior vena cava. Surg Gynecol Obstet 1983;156:659–660.
31. Coit DG, Turnbull ADM. Long-term central vascular access through the gonadal vein. Surg Gynecol Obstet 1992;175:362–364.
32. Boddie AW Jr. Translumbar catheterization of the inferior vena cava for long-term angioaccess. Surg Gynecol Obstet 1989;168:55–56.
33. Kenney PR, Dorfman GS, Denny DF Jr. Percutaneous inferior vena cava cannultation for long-term parenteral nutrition. Surgery 1985;97:602–604.
34. Torosian MH, Meranze S, Mullen JL, McLean G. Central venous access with occlusive superior central venous thrombosis. Ann Surg 1986;203:30–33.

6

Thrombotic and Occlusive Complications of Long-Term Venous Access: Diagnosis, Management, and Prophylaxis

H. Richard Alexander

Catheter Occlusion and Persistent Withdrawal
    Occlusion
        Catheter Occlusion
        Withdrawal Occlusion
        Treatment
Catheter-Related Venous Thrombosis
        Incidence and Etiology
        Diagnosis
        Treatment
        Prophylaxis
References

The timely diagnosis and treatment of catheter occlusion or catheter-related venous thrombosis are important to maximize the possibility of restoring catheter function, extend the life of the catheter, and minimize the consequences of progressive symptomatic venous thrombosis.

Catheter Occlusion and Persistent Withdrawal Occlusion

Catheter Occlusion

The inability to infuse fluids through the catheter is frequently first encountered by the nurse prior to initiating a cycle of infusional therapy and can be a manifestation of catheter tip migration or malposition with kinking, luminal occlusion by blood clot or precipitation of drug solutions, an extensive fibrin sheath around the catheter tip, or catheter tip abutment against the vein wall.[1-4] The presence of luminal clots has been reported in up to 93% of Hickman catheters and in up to 50% of Groshong catheters.[5,6] The development of a luminal blood clot is presumably due to the reflux and stasis of blood into the catheter lumen. Occasionally, a catheter may be occluded because of catheter "pinch-off."[7] This occurs when the catheter has been inserted too medially under the clavicle, adjacent to the costoclavicular ligament, and is pinched by the scissoring action of the clavicle on the first rib (Figure 6-1). If the catheter is subjected to repetitive pinching over time it can shear off completely. Cassidy reported the findings of 77 venographic studies performed on patients with malfunctioning long-term venous access catheters.[2] The relative frequency of noninfectious complications in patients with Hickman catheters is shown in Table 6-1.

Catheter occlusion is easily diagnosed after attempts to restore patency with a syringe and dilute heparin solution are unsuccessful.

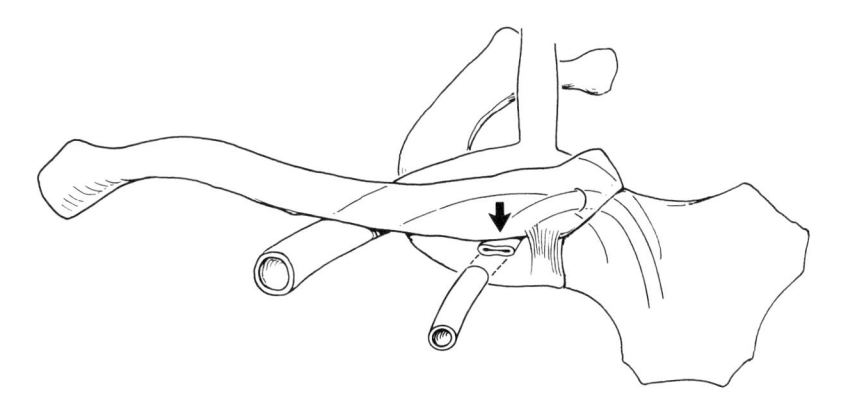

FIGURE 6-1. Schematic illustration of possible pinching effect of the first rib and clavicle on a long-term venous access catheter inserted medially adjacent to or through the costoclavicular ligament.

TABLE 6-1
Noninfectious Complications Associated with Hickman Long-Term Vascular Access Catheters

Venographic Findings	Hickman (N = 117)
Fibrin sheath	24
Catheter migration	8
Catheter constriction by a suture	6
Catheter tip abutment against vein wall	2
Contrast extravasation	3
Malpositioned catheter tips	2
Catheter leak	1
Complete catheter occlusion	0
Venous thrombosis	6
No abnormality	2

From Cassidy FP Jr, Zajko AB, Bron KM, Reilly JJ Jr, Peitzman AB, Steed DL. Noninfectious complications of long-term central venous catheters: radiologic evaluation and management. AJR 1987;149:671–675. Used with permission.

The next step should be to obtain a chest x-ray (or appropriate film if the catheter is in a subdiaphragmatic position) to rule out kinking or malposition. If the catheter appears to be in the correct position and there is no change from previous x-ray films then migration or kinking can be ruled out. Stokes has measured resistance to flow (R) through Hickman or Broviac catheters and found it to be a sensitive and simple test to diagnose catheter obstruction. Decreases in R correlate well with return of catheter function after thrombolytic therapy.[8] This diagnostic tool may simplify the evaluation and treatment of partially obstructed catheters by reducing the number of radiographic studies necessary to evaluate an occluded catheter.

One completely preventable cause of catheter occlusion is intraluminal precipitation caused by incompatible mixtures of drugs/solutions (eg, Dilantin/D_5W). Prevention is often the only course of action, because once the drug crystals have lodged within the catheter lumen they are extremely difficult to dissolve. If drug precipitate is highly suspected, the application of warm soaks over the catheter tunnel may help reverse the crystallization.

Catheter occlusions may be attributed to precipitates of poorly soluble fluid components, such as the calcium salts in total parenteral nutrition (TPN). Although thrombolytic agents are ineffective in these circumstances, catheter patency can be restored if the solubility of the fluid components is increased, eg, by lowering the pH by using 0.1N hydrochloric acid (HCl). Because of its safety, efficacy, and low cost (especially when compared with device replacement), HCl should be considered as an additional agent to clear an obstructed catheter of unknown etiology.[9] Occlusions that are caused by lipid-containing solutions have been successfully cleared by the use of a 70% solution of ethanol in sterile water.[10]

Withdrawal Occlusion

If one can infuse through the device but not aspirate this is termed catheter withdrawal occlusion. If this phenomenon is encountered early after insertion it is most likely secondary to the catheter being inserted too medially so that it is slightly compressed as it traverses between the first rib and clavicle. Under these conditions, the lumen itself may collapse secondary to the negative pressure generated during as aspiration attempt (Figure 6-1). If withdrawal occlusion is encountered at some later time in the life of the catheter, this has been attributed to the development of a fibrin sheath around the tip of the catheter acting as a flap valve which does not interfere with infusion but does prevent aspiration.[11] The incidence of catheter withdrawal occlusion has been reported to occur in up to 80% of patients with long-term venous access catheters.[4] Another possibility is that the tip has abutted against a vein wall such that any attempts to aspirate will result in collapse of the vein against the lumen. Although it is extremely unpredictable, anecdotal experience with asking the patient to valsalva, cough, deep breathe, raise arms over his head, or lie in different positions (left or right lateral or in Trendelenberg) occasionally have been successful in restoring the ability to aspirate blood. Even with persistent withdrawal occlusion a catheter can still be used for infusional therapy. However, venipuncture will be required for blood tests. The decision to replace the catheter on the basis of withdrawal occlusion alone is not typically indicated unless the difficulty in repeated venous access is enormous.

Treatment

If a catheter has been found to have migrated and is malpositioned or kinked as the basis for catheter occlusion the management may involve an interventional radiology procedure to place the catheter tip in the appropriate position.[2] Catheters that have flipped into the contralateral subclavian vein or internal jugular vein may be repositioned in this fashion. This should be attempted only if one is confident on the basis of plain x-ray or contrast study that the catheter is still intravenous. Occasionally a catheter will withdraw partially from the vein and an x-ray film will demonstrate the catheter tip in the subclavian vein and the remaining part coiled in the subcutaneous tissue beneath the clavicle. In this instance the catheter should be removed and replaced as the possibility that the catheter will migrate further cannot be excluded.

After excluding malposition or a large catheter-related venous thrombosis as the etiology of an occluded catheter or persistent withdrawal occlusion, attempts to restore patency with a variety of thrombolytic agents can be very successful (Table 6-2). Although there is some possibility of embolizing a small luminal clot into the lungs, the

TABLE 6-2
Success of Thrombolytic Therapy for Occluded Venous Access Device: Selected Reports

Author	Agent	Indications	Dose	Duration of Treatment	Outcome
Atkinson et al[17]	t-PA	O*	2 mg/2 mL	4 h	80%‡ success (mean 1.5 doses)
Kersen et al[13]	Urokinase	O	5000 U/h	16–72 h	22/25 resolved
Tschirhart and Rao[11]	Urokinase	PWO†	250,000 U in 150 mL D$_s$W	90 min	10/11 cleared
Lawson et al[12]	Urokinase	O	5000 U/mL 0.3–0.4 mL	5–60 min	98.6% success§
Wachs[15]	Urokinase	O	5000 U in 1 mL	30 min	98% success‖
Hurtubise et al[16]	Urokinase Varidase	O	5000 U/mL 250 U/mL (streptokinase)	0.3–0.6 mL ×30 min	77% cleared within 22 min 100% overall

*O = occlusion.
†Persistent withdrawal occlusion.
‡Had previously failed to clear with urokinase.
§Most were not Silastic catheters.
‖Pediatric patients.

clinical consequences do not appear significant. Tschirhart has reported on the success of using a short urokinase infusion in the management of persistent withdrawal occlusion (PWO) in totally implanted ports.[11] Of 42 cancer patients with totally implanted ports, 8 (19%) developed 11 episodes of PWO. Ipsilateral venograms confirmed the presence of a fibrin or thrombotic sheath extending from the entrance site of the catheter into the vein and extending from 1 to 5 cm beyond the catheter tip. The PWO occurred from 18 to 65 days after implantation and had been present for up to 4 months, suggesting that long-standing PWO can be successfully treated. Administration of urokinase, 250,000 U in 150 mL of D$_5$W, infused over 90 minutes produced complete remission of withdrawal occlusion in more than 90% of catheters. Withdrawal occlusion recurred three times but not in any patient who had documented complete resolution of the sheath.

Lawson et al have reported a 98.6% success rate in restoring patency in more than 1600 occluded central venous catheters which were primarily silicone elastomer or Teflon.[12] Urokinase, 5000 U/mL, was instilled into the occluded catheter with a tuberculin syringe in a volume estimated to be equal to or slightly less than the volume of the catheter (0.2 to 0.4 mL). Every 5 minutes attempts were made to aspirate the catheter and after 1 hour the urokinase treatment was repeated if necessary. Kersen has reported that 22 of 25 patients with both external and implanted devices with venogram confirmation of catheter occulusion were successfully treated with a urokinase infusion, 5000 U/h, for 16 to 72 hours.[13] In this series there were a small number of patients with coexisting subclavian vein thrombosis and urokinase treatment restored catheter patency even when the subclavian thrombosis was not completely resolved. The time course of catheter occlusion was extremely variable, occurring from 1 to 25 months after catheter placement. Others have used 2 mL of urokinase, 5000 U/mL, infused and left in the catheter for 30 minutes to 2 hours.[14]

The utility of urokinase for declotting indwelling venous catheters in pediatric patients has also been reported. In the pediatric patient population the ability to restore catheter function appears particularly important as replacement of a catheter in an infant involves a small but real surgical risk. In 101 of 103 episodes of partial or total catheter occlusion patency was restored with urokinase.[15] The regimen utilized was 5000 U/mL of urokinase instilled into each lumen. For implanted ports 2 mL were infused to accommodate the volume of extension tubing. In this series one third of patients required a second dose to restore patency. There were no untoward effects of urokinase administration.

Alternately, a commercially available combination of streptokinase with streptodornase can be administered in a volume equal to the estimated internal volume of the catheter (approximately 0.6 mL for subclavian catheters).[16] Saline is added to the stock vial to produce a final concentration of 250 U/mL of streptokinase. Hurtuboise et al have reported the successful use of streptokinase in 266 occluded catheters.[16] Patency was restored with a single dose on average in 22 minutes in 77% and in an additional 23% a second or third dose restored patency on average in 45 minutes.

There have been no hemorrhagic complications attributed to the use of urokinase or streptokinase in these studies.[13,14,16] Hurtubise monitored a variety of coagulation parameters in 14 patients receiving either streptokinase or urokinase and saw no changes compared to baseline (Table 6-3). It does not appear that fibrinolytic agents used in

TABLE 6-3
Fibrinolytic Therapy of Occluded Venous Catheters Does Not Alter Coagulation Parameters

	Platelet (mm³)	Partial Thromboplastin Time (s)	Prothrombin Time (s)	Prothrombin Time (s)	Fibrinogen (mg/dL)
Baseline, h	(13–346)* 25	(21.5–47.5) 30.7	(10.1–12.7) 11.8	(10.8–12.4) 11.5	(40–740) 385
2	(8–246) 32	(23.6–45.3) 27.5	(10.1–14.2) 11.6	(10.8–12.4) 11.4	(105–600) 450
4	(6–367) 37	(21.6–42.6) 28.5	(10.5–14.2) 11.0	(10.8–12.5) 11.3	(115–720) 410
6	(5–257) 34	(21.9–35.9) 27.8	(10.5–14.7) 11.6	(10.8–12.5) 11.4	(120–700) 400
24	(11–410) 43	(23.3–50.2) 29.0	(11.0–16) 11.9	(10.9–12.3) 11.7	(125–640) 435

*Numbers in parentheses indicate the range.
From Hurtubise MR, Bottino JC, Lawson M, McCredie KB. Restoring patency of occluded central venous catheters. Arch Surg 1980;115:212–213. Used with permission.

TABLE 6-4
Fibrinolytic Therapy with t-PA for Occluded Central Venous Catheters Does Not Alter Coagulation Profiles

	Platelets (mm³)	PT (s)	PTT (s)	Fibrinogen (mg/dL)	Plasminogen (mg/dL)	FDP (mg/dL)
Pretreatment	300–500*	10.9–13.1	24–31	270–1040	120–135	8–16
	(400)	(11.9)	(29)	(320)	(124)	(8)
Posttreatment	400–520	11.2–12.4	25–41	225–520	118	8–32
	(496)	(11.7)	(39)	(310)		(8)

*Indicates range. Numbers in parentheses denote median.
From Atkinson JB, Bagnall HA, Gomperts E. Investigational use of tissue plasminogen activator (t-PA) for occluded central venous catheters. JPEN 1990;14:310–311. Used with permission.

these doses have any effect on clotting parameters even in the presence of preexisting clotting indices. The need to intensively monitor these parameters during treatment does not appear essential.

Tissue plasminogen activator (t-PA) has also been used successfully in the treatment of occluded central venous catheters that failed to clear with urokinase.[17] Atkinson et al reported that five of six occluded chronic indwelling venous catheters were successfully treated with a 4-hour instillation of 2 mg/2 mL of t-PA. Up to three doses were used without complication. The failure of one catheter to clear was attributed to malposition of the tip. At this dose there were no bleeding or hemorrhagic complications (Table 6-4).

In summary, catheter occlusion or persistent withdrawal occlusion can be managed effectively and safely with instillation of a variety of fibrinolytic agents. In most series addressing the issue of catheter occlusion, those rare failures of urokinase to restore patency appear to be in patients with phenytoin or diazepam precipitation in the catheter.[12,15,18]

Catheter-Related Venous Thrombosis

The presence of a chronic indwelling venous catheter in the subclavian or other vein and the associated intimal injury at the insertion site predisposes patients to the development of venous thromboses. Central venous catheters may account for about 40% of all deep venous thromboses of the upper extremity.[19] Pulmonary embolism occurs in approximately 12% of patients with venous thromboses of the subclavian or axillary vein.[19] The fact that many subclavian vein thromboses remain asymptomatic may be secondary to several factors including the presence of extensive venous collaterals in the upper extremity that minimize the hemodynamic effect of an intramural thrombus and that hydrostatic forces favor venous drainage from the upper extremity to a much greater extent than the lower extremity.[20] After anticoagulation treatment, the short- and long-term sequelae of upper central venous thrombosis such as secondary thrombophlebitis or chronic extremity edema appear minimal.[21] Although some patients with asymptomatic venous thromboses detected on screening phlebography have been treated with catheter removal and observation alone,[22] this may not represent the optimal approach. It has been shown that sleeve thromboses can break off and embolize during catheter removal and produce clinically significant[23,24] or even fatal[25] pulmonary emboli. Once a diagnosis of catheter-related venous thrombosis is made prompt treatment is indicated (see section on treatment).

Incidence and Etiology

Catheter-related venous thrombosis has been reported to occur from 4% to 40% of patients by clinical assessment or autopsy.[22,23,26–28] Chastre demonstrated that slightly more than 60% of critically ill patients with indwelling pulmonary artery catheters inserted through the internal jugular vein developed asymptomatic venous thromboses within 6 days of catheterization, suggesting that the actual incidence in patients with long term indwelling subclavian vein catheters may be higher than reported, as many thromboses are clinically inapparent.[29] In this study the development of venous thrombosis was associated with the presence and duration of a decreased cardiac index, making it not entirely applicable to the population with indwelling venous catheters.

Subsequent studies in cancer patients with long-term venous catheters have confirmed the high incidence of thrombosis in this group of patients. Lokich and Becker, in a combined retrospective and prospective study of 42 cancer patients receiving infusional chemotherapy for advanced malignancy, found a 42% incidence of subclavian vein thrombosis.[22] The manifestation of trombosis and the time to onset after catheter insertion was highly variable. Thromboses were detected from 5 to 270 days after catheter insertion (mean of 30 days). About one half of patients initially presented with mild symptoms including neck or arm pain and jugular venous distension. Thromboses that present as partial or complete vena caval syndrome with massive arm edema were rare. Predisposing factors for the development of thrombosis included hypercoagulability (decreased antithrombin III levels), mediastinal tumors with possible venous flow abnormalities, and suboptimal catheter care routine. In another series of 168 patients with solid tumors evaluated clinically or at autopsy, Anderson et al[26] have reported an overall thrombosis rate of 17%. The actual incidence may have been higher as only one quarter of patients underwent autopsy. Interestingly, patients with adenocarcinoma of the lung had a significantly higher rate of thrombosis (45%) compared to patients with squamous carcinomas of lung and other sites, indicating that tumor histology is a risk factor for the development of thrombosis (Table 6-5). The time to development of thrombosis was highly variable, occurring from 20 to 240 days after catheter insertion.

Brismar et al have reported a study of 60 catheterizations in 53

TABLE 6-5
Incidence of Catheter-Related Venous Thrombosis in Patients with Solid Tumors

Primary Tumor	No. of Patients with External Catheters	Current Status Alive	Current Status Dead	Thrombosis No. (%)
Lung cancer				
Squamous	46	6	40	7 (15)
Adenocarcinoma	20	5	15	9 (45)
Large cell	5	0	5	2 (40)
Head and neck	56	21	35	5 (9)
Esophagus	24	6	18	4 (17)
Miscellaneous	9	5	4	0 (0)

From Anderson AJ, Krasnow SH, Boyer MW, et al. Thrombosis: the major Hickman catheter complication in patients with solid tumor. Chest 1989;95:71–75. Used with permission.

patients with a variety of benign diagnoses for the administration of TPN.[23] In this study, the incidence of catheter-related thrombosis appeared to increase with the duration of catheterization. However, other studies have not observed this trend[22,26,28] and Haire et al have reported that 60% of catheter related venous thromboses developed within 14 days of catheter placement and 70% within 1 month (Figure 6-2).[30] Haire's study of 168 patients undergoing bone marrow transplantation and 49 other patients receiving high dose chemotherapy for a variety of hematologic malignancies showed that the development of thrombi occurred earlier in patients undergoing bone marrow transplantation although the overall incidence at 100 days after catheterization was comparable.

Although others have shown that the development of catheter related venous thrombosis is related to hypercoagulability,[22] Haire's study, using linear regression analysis, identified a higher platelet count as a predisposing factor toward thrombosis (Figure 6-3). This suggests that in the setting of venous intimal injury and a long-term intravascular catheter, platelets may be important in the etiology of thrombosis formation and that antiplatelet therapy may be useful in prophylaxis against catheter-related thrombi. In addition, the development of venous thrombosis was higher in patients receiving bilateral venous catheters comparted with unilateral catheters. Jacobson and Brismas have reported that the incidence of catheter related venous thrombosis in patients receiving total parenteral nutrition is higher with a blood hemoglobin level greater than 12.5 g/dL.[31]

In summary, the incidence of catheter-related venous thrombosis is variable but may occur most frequently soon after placement of the catheter when venous intimal injury is new. In contrast to primary subclavian vein thrombosis, the possibility of pulmonary embolism or progression to complete vena cava syndrome is not inconsequential

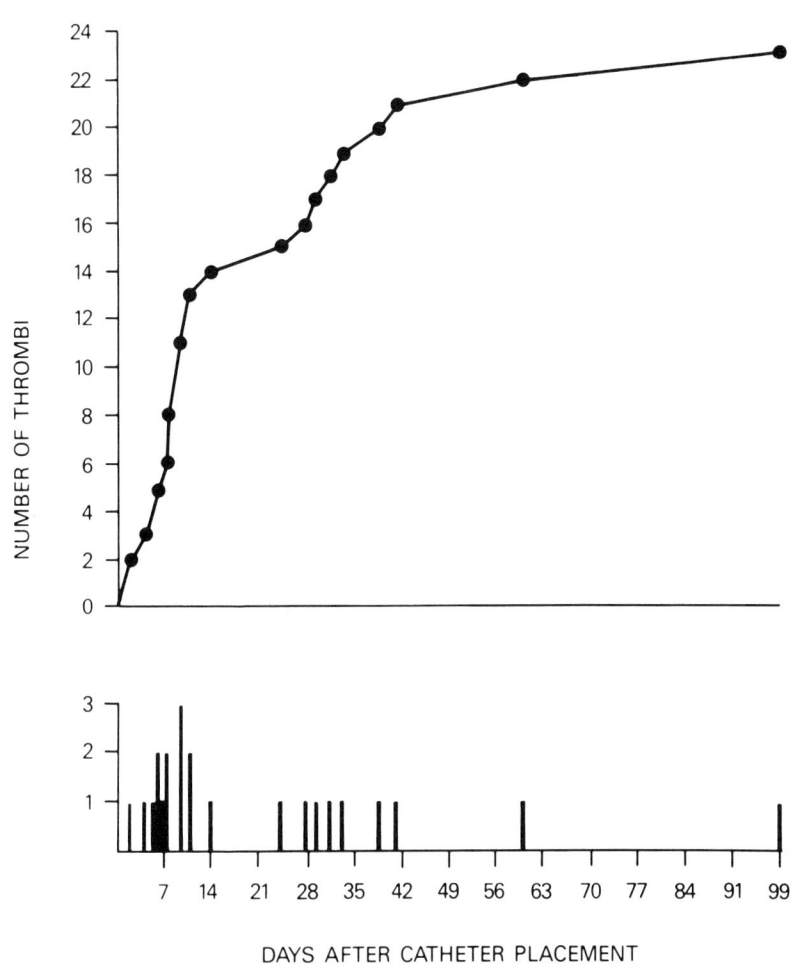

FIGURE 6-2. Incidence and time course of long-term venous access catheter-related thoracic venous thrombosis in 225 adult cancer patients. Slightly over half of the thromboses developed within 2 weeks after catheter placement and two thirds developed within 1 month of catheter placement. Reproduced from Haire WD, Lieberman RP, Edney J, et al. Hickman catheterinduced thoracic vein thrombosis. Cancer 1990;66:900–908. Used with permission.

and warrants prompt attention. Risk factors for the development of catheter related venous thrombosis include solid tumors, particularly adenocarcinoma of the lung, mediastinal tumors, low flow states, hypercoagulability, and bilateral vs unilateral venous access lines. Factors not associated with catheter-related venous thrombosis include age, sex, history of a previous venous access catheter, or technique of placement.[28]

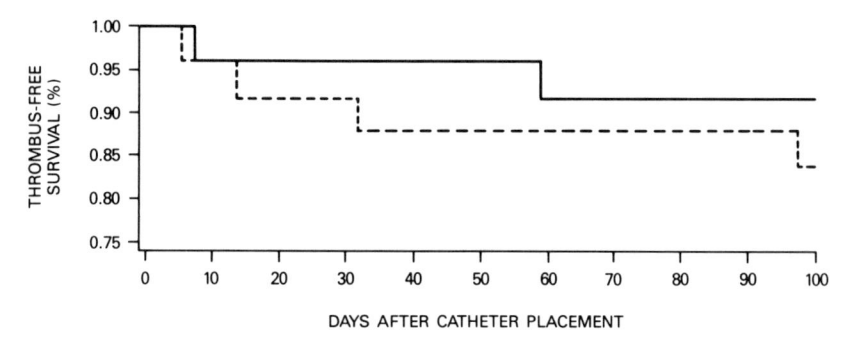

FIGURE 6-3. Thrombus-free survival in patients with long-term venous access catheters who have platelet counts greater than or equal to 150,000 (*solid line*) or less than 150,000 (*dashed line*) at the time of catheter insertion. The difference in thrombus-free survival between the groups is significant. Modified from Haire WD, Lieberman RP, Edney J, et al. Hickman catheter-induced thoracic vein thrombosis. Cancer 1990;66:900–908. Used with permission.

Diagnosis

The major contribution of the studies published to date addressing catheter-related subclavian vein thrombosis have been to define the incidence, presentation, and risk factors associated with catheter-related venous thrombosis. An appreciation of these factors may then be used to influence more effectively the timing, duration, and nature of prophylactic or therapeutic treatment of venous thrombosis.

Patients who develop symptoms compatible with subclavian vein thrombosis such as arm swelling, pain, and evidence of collateral venous flow on the chest wall may be evaluated with peripheral venography,[2,29] duplex Doppler sonography, or computed tomography (CT) scan[20,32] (Table 6-6). There are characteristic findings on chest x-ray film that may lead one to suspect venous thrombosis but the findings are not specific and a normal chest x-ray film does not eliminate the possibility of a thrombus.[33] The use of contrast instilled through the in situ catheter can demonstrate both distal thrombosis and a fibrin sheath. However, no information about the proximal extent of the thrombus or the degree of subclavian vein thrombosis can be obtained.

Falk and Smith have reported on the successful use of duplex Doppler sonography to diagnose upper extremity thoracic inlet venous thrombosis.[32] With the use of Doppler sonography normal vessels demonstrate a characteristic sharp echogenic pattern and flow signals that vary with respiratory variation. In contrast, thrombosed vessels have poorly defined echogenic lumens and absent or diminished flow patterns. In 18 patients with CT- or venogram-documented ve-

TABLE 6-6
Methods for Diagnosing Catheter Related Venous Thrombosis

Technique	Possible Findings	Disadvantage/Advantage
Chest x-ray	Enlargement of superior vena cava, new pleural effusions, dilated collateral veins (ie, azygos, left superior intercostal)	Nonspecific Not sensitive Noninvasive
Color-flow Doppler ultrasound	Thrombus is an echogenic filling defect, characteristic signal absent or abnormal, loss of respiratory variability in flow	Noninvasive Portable, cannot detect partial thrombosis, cannot image intrathoracic veins
Chest CT	Opacification of venous lumens altered, demonstrate collaterals, distinguish compression from thrombus, can identify site of obstruction	Does not demonstrate small nonocclusive thrombi
MRI	Characteristic signal of thrombus, possible perivenous edema	Limited availability, expensive
Venography	Best resolution of venous anatomy including patency, location of thrombus, and presence of collaterals	Ipsilateral forearm venous access may be difficult

nous thrombosis duplex Doppler sonography was diagnostic in all cases, with only one false-positive test. It has the advantage of portability and high patient acceptance. Bolz has reported using intravascular ultrasonography in 12 patients with indwelling catheters to diagnose catheter-related venous thrombosis. All patients were cannulated via the femoral vein and the studies lasted on average of 7.5 minutes.[34] Although two central venous thrombi and one malpositioned catheter were diagnosed with intravascular ultrasound, it is not clear what advantages this study may have in this setting over other established diagnostic modalities.

Although contrast enhanced CT or magnetic resonance imaging (MRI) are very sensitive, they have the disadvantages of expense and occasional difficulties in availability. They may be the test of choice for patients with suspected septic venous thrombi as additional information regarding surrounding inflammatory infiltration or gas within the thrombi can be obtained.[35] Fever has been reported as a finding of venous thrombosis even in the absence of documented infection.[21]

The standard diagnostic test for venous thrombosis remains venography. In some patients ipsilateral forearm venous access may be difficult. However, the study does provide a detailed assessment of the location and extent of intramural thrombosis, the flow patterns through the vein or collaterals, and information about the more central venous anatomy.

Treatment

One of the main unresolved issues that dominates the management approach of catheter-related subclavian vein thromboses centers around the role of catheter removal after a thrombosis has been diagnosed. In the past, catheter removal, systemic anticoagulation with heparin, and subsequent coumadin treatment has been a fairly standard approach for catheter-related thrombosis.[21,22] Although removal of the offending catheter is intuitive, recent reports have demonstrated highly successful treatment with anticoagulation or thrombolytic agents while the catheter remains in situ.[28,36–39] Initial supportive measures include arm elevation and analgesia for pain.

The use of systemic streptokinase for refractory catheter-related subclavian vein thrombosis was originally reported by Rubenstein and Creger.[40] In this case report the catheter was removed but venography showed extension of the clot on heparin therapy. Treatment with a loading dose of septokinase 250,000 U intravenously followed by 100,000 U/h for 72 hours resulted in complete clot dissolution. However, a nonfatal pulmonary embolism may have been precipitated by treatment with streptokinase. Two subsequent small series of patients with both catheter-related and non-catheter-related axillary-subclavian vein thromboses have reported successful treatment with systemic streptokinase in a comparable manner have also been reported.[22,41] Hemorrhagic complications with the use of systemic streptokinase in these series was not inconsequential and close monitoring of the patient is essential.

Fraschini et al[39] have reported the results of local urokinase infusion for the treatment of catheter-related venous thrombosis in 35 patients. Urokinase was administered intravenously as a loading dose of 500 U/kg followed by a dose of 500 to 2000 U/kg/h for an interval of 1 to 4 days. Patients were assessed with serial venograms daily. Theoretically, the local infusion of urokinase to the site of thrombus should provide the maximum therapeutic effect with the minimum toxicity (Figure 6-4). To achieve this catheters were withdrawn partially so that the tip was positioned adjacent to the thrombus or an ipsilateral peripheral intravenous catheter was inserted. The advantage of using a second peripheral catheter is that the long-term venous catheter can potentially be used if complete clot lysis can be achieved (Figure 6-5). Complete lysis of thrombi occurred in 25 of 30 patients whose clots were directly infused with urokinase and only two had recurrence of thrombi (Table 6-7). All patients with partial lysis had recurrent thrombi. The results of this report indicate that the ability to successfully treat a subclavian vein thrombosis with thrombolytic therapy is related to the duration of symptoms. Dissolution of thrombi was achieved in more than 90% of patients who had a short (less than 1 week) interval of symptoms compared to only 56% of patients with symptoms lasting longer than 1 week. This suggests that once a diagnosis of subclavian vein thrombosis is made, particularly if symptoms

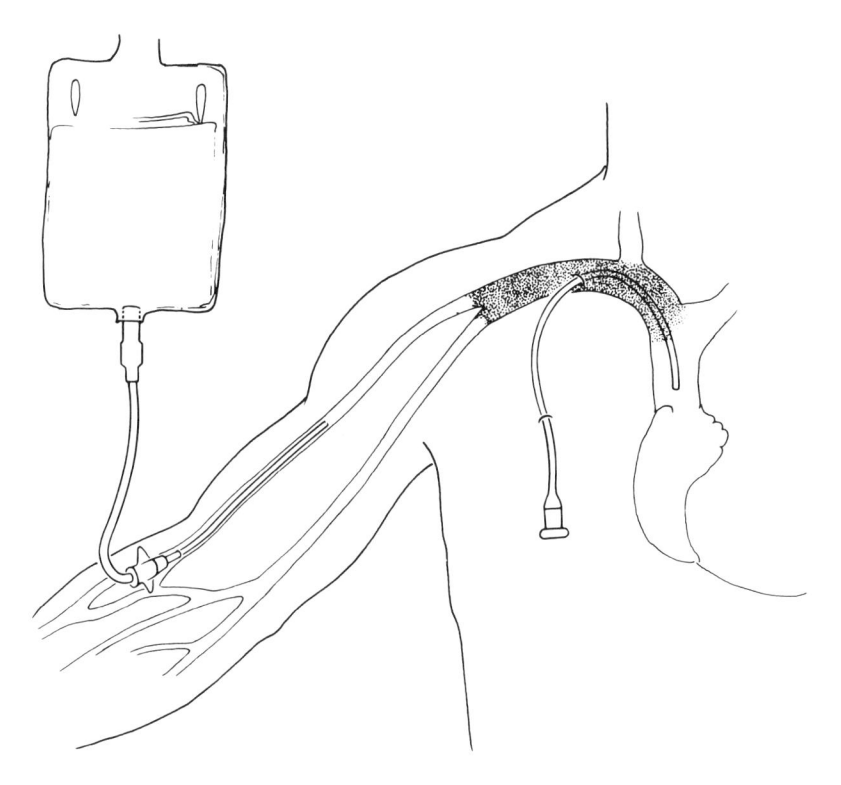

FIGURE 6-4. The local infusion of thrombolytic therapy ideally should be directed through an ipsilateral forearm vein to the site of the thrombus.

are present, prompt treatment is indicated. Hemorrhagic complications with local infusion urokinase were observed in almost half of the patients but were minor in nature.

The efficacy and safety of urokinase therapy for catheter-induced venous thrombi in infants and children have also been reported. This is a particularly important issue as the preservation of catheter function will obviate the need for repeated anesthetics for catheter replacement. Curnow et al reported that 12 cases of documented venous thrombosis occurred in patients ranging from 6 weeks to 43 months of age.[42] With all patients being monitored in the intensive care unit, urokinase was infused through the catheter using a loading dose of 4400 U/kg intravenously over 10 minutes followed by a continuous infusion of 4400 U/kg/h for 4 hours. If residual thrombus was identified, the protocol was repeated first using 6600 U/kg followed by 8800 U/kg if necessary. In 10 of 12 patients a single course of urokinase resulted in complete resolution of thrombus as assessed by catheter venography or two-dimensional echocardiography. Catheters were preserved in nine patients. There were no major complications.

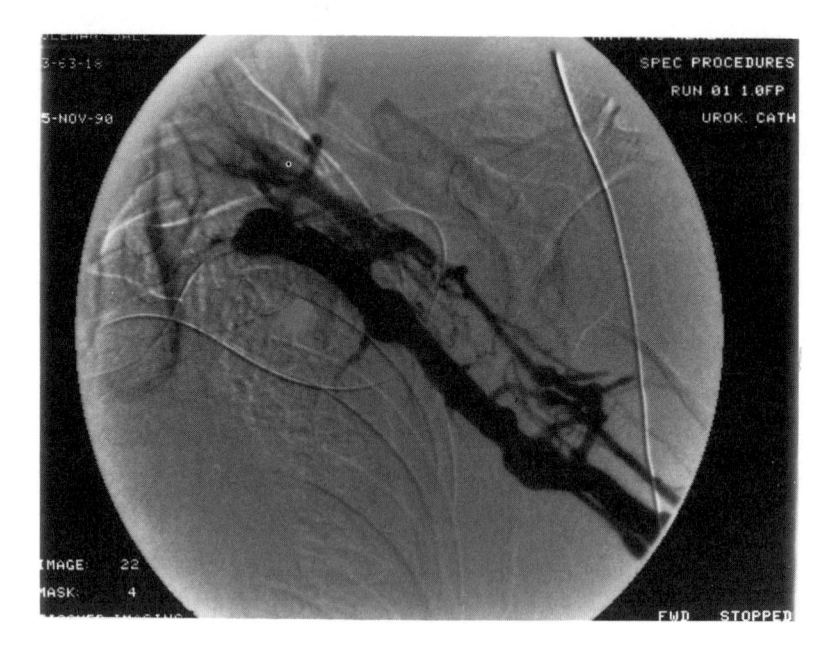

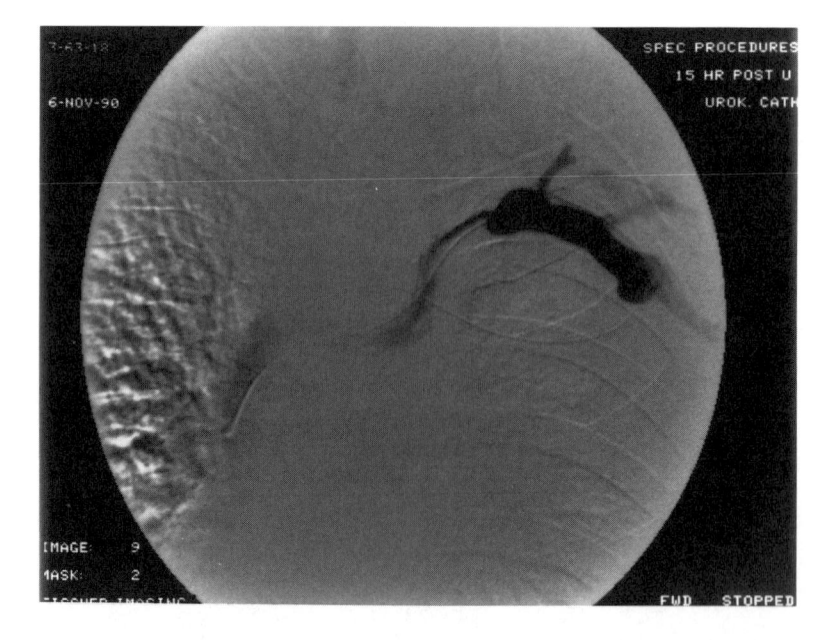

FIGURE 6-5. Catheter related subclavian thrombosis (*top*) with nearly complete occlusion of the vein. After a 15 hour infusion of urokinase through an ipsilateral forearm vein there is partial resolution of the thrombus (*bottom*). Two weeks after completion of a 24-hour infusion of thrombolytic therapy the subclavian vein shows wide patency with no evidence of intravascular thrombus (*next page*). The catheter was fully functional at the completion of treatment.

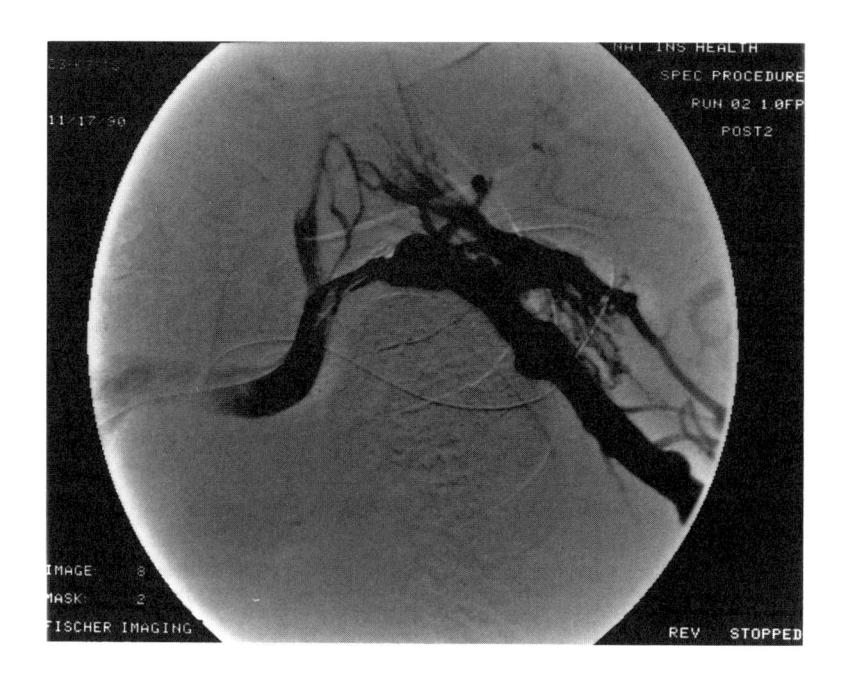

FIGURE 6-5. *Continued*

Prophylaxis

Several studies have reported prophylactic treatment of patients with indwelling venous catheters in an attempt to reduce the incidence of thrombus formation. Fabri et al have reported that patients receiving TPN through polyvinyl chloride central venous catheters with low-dose heparin added to the TPN solution will reduce the incidence of asymptomatic catheter-related thrombosis to one third that observed in patients without heparin.[43] In an older study of central venous

TABLE 6-7

Response of Catheter-Related Venous Thrombi Treated by Direct Infusion with Urokinase

Extent of Thrombus Directly Infused	No. of Patients	Response Complete Lysis	Partial Lysis	No Lysis
Entire thrombus	23	18	1	4
Portion	7	7	0	0
Total	30	25	1	4

From Fraschini G, Jadeja J, Lawson M, Holmes FA, Carrasco HC, Wallace S. Local infusion of urokinase for the lysis of thrombosis associated with permanent central venous catheters in cancer patients. J Clin Oncol 1987;5:672–678. Used with permission.

catheters inserted for parenteral nutrition, Brismar demonstrated that intravenous heparin, 5000 U/6 h, administered through the catheter reduced the incidence of catheter-associated thrombotic complications.[44] In patients with indwelling pulmonary artery catheters for hemodynamic monitoring during cardiopulmonary bypass, the use of heparin-bonded catheters significantly reduced the incidence of thrombus formation on the catheter.[45]

A prospective randomized trial evaluating the use of daily low-dose prophylactic warfarin in adult cancer patients with long-term indwelling venous catheters has been reported by Bern et al.[46] Most patients had a diagnosis of solid tumor malignancy and represented a group at high risk for catheter-related venous thrombosis as evidenced by the fact that almost 40% of the control arm developed a thrombotic complication within 90 days of catheter insertion. The incidence of venous thrombosis, the majority of which were symptomatic, was significantly reduced from 38% in untreated controls to 9.5% in patients receiving low-dose warfarin (1 mg/day) (Figure 6-6). Virtually all thromboses in both groups were symptomatic; the addi-

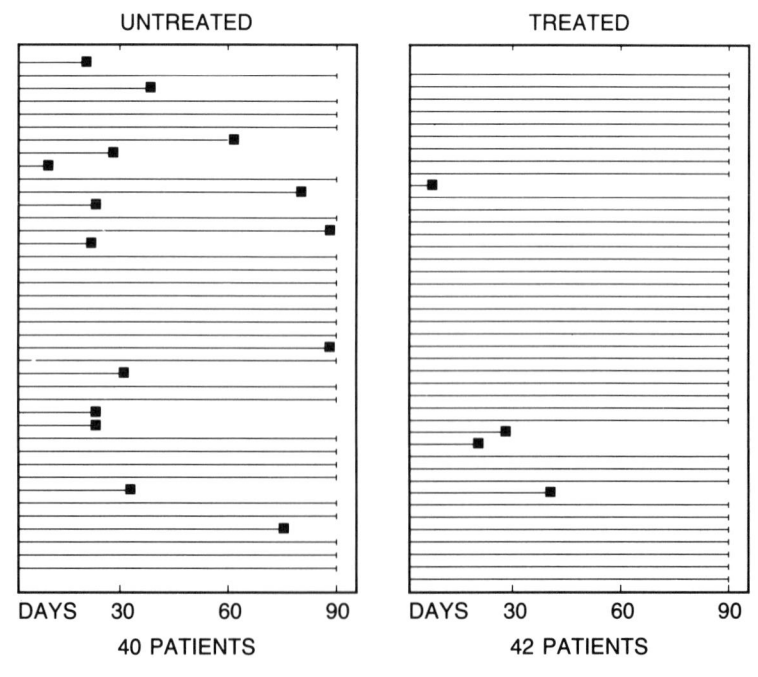

FIGURE 6-6. Number and timing of catheter-related venous thromboses in a prospective randomized trial of adult cancer patients receiving or not receiving low-dose warfarin daily after catheter insertion. The number of thromboses is significantly less in patients receiving warfarin versus placebo. Reproduced from Bern MM, Lokich JJ, Wallach SR, et al. Very low doses of warfarin can prevent thrombosis in central venous catheters. Ann Intern Med 1990;112:423–428. Used with permission.

tion of warfarin had no effect on coagulation parameters and was well tolerated. The findings of this study indicate that the incidence of catheter-related thromboses can be substantially reduced in patients at risk for thromboses and methods to more accurately identify which patients are a high risk and might benefit from prophylactic treatment will allow more judicious use of this approach.

References

1. Lawson M. Partial occlusion of indwelling central venous catheters. JIN 1991;14:157–159.
2. Cassidy FP Jr, Zajko AB, Bron KM, Reilly JJ Jr, Peitzman AB, Steed DL. Noninfectious complications of long-term central venous catheters: radiologic evaluation and management. AJR 1987;149:671–675.
3. Lazarus HM, Lowder JN, Herzig RH. Occlusion and infection in Broviac catheters during intensive cancer therapy. Cancer 1983;52:2342–2348.
4. Peters WR, Bush WH Jr. The development of fibrin sheath on indwelling venous catheters. Surg Gynecol Obstet 1973;137:43–47.
5. Anderson AJ, Krawnow SH, Boyer MW, et al. Hickman catheter clots: a common occurrence despite daily heparin flushing. Cancer Treat Rep 1987;71:651–653.
6. Anderson AJ, Krasnow SH, Boyer MW, Wadleigh RG, Cohen MH. Clots can frequently be aspirated from Groshong catheters. Am Assoc Cancer Res 1988;29:A907:228. (Abstract)
7. Aitken DR, Minton JP. The "pinch-off sign": a warning of impending problems with permanent subclavian catheters. Am J Surg 1984;148:633.
8. Stokes DC, Rao BN, Mirro J Jr, et al. Early detection and simplified management of obstructed Hickman and Broviac catheters. J Pediatr Surg 1989;24:257–262.
9. Shulman RJ, Reed T, Pitre D, et al. Use of hydrochloric acid to clear obstructed central venous catheters. JPEN 12: 1988;509–510.
10. Pennington CR, Pithie AD. Ethanol lock in the management of catheter occlusion. JPEN 1987;11:507–508.
11. Tschirhart JM, Rao MK. Mechanism and management of persistent withdrawal occlusion. Am Surg 1988;54:326–328.
12. Lawson M, Bottino JC, Hurtubise MR, McCredie KB. The use of urokinase to restore the patency of occluded central venous catheters. Am J Intraven Ther Clin Nutr 1982;5:29–32.
13. Kersen C, DiStetano A, Blumenschein G, Larson A, Kelly JP, Firstenberg B. Treatment of vascular access catheter occlusion with urokinase infusion. Am Assoc Cancer Res 1988;29:A908: 228. (Abstract)
14. Gillies H, Rogers HJ, Johnston J, Harper PG, Rudge CJ. Is repeated flushing of Hickman catheters necessary? Br Med J 1985;290:1708.

15. Wachs T. Urokinase administration in pediatric patients with occluded central venous catheters. JIN 1990;13:100–102.
16. Hurtubise MR, Bottino JC, Lawson M, McCredie KB. Restoring patency of occluded central venous catheters. Arch Surg 1980;115:212–213.
17. Atkinson JB, Bagnall HA, Gomperts E. Investigational use of tissue plasminogen activator (t-PA) for occluded central venous catheters. JPEN 1990;14:310–311.
18. Boku T, Nakane Y, Okusa T, et al. Strategy for lymphadenectomy of gastric cancer. Surgery 1989;105:585–592.
19. Horattas MC, Wright DJ, Fenton AH, et al. Changing concepts of deep venous thrombosis of the upper extremity-report of a series and review of the literature. Surgery 1988;104:561–567.
20. Wechsler RJ, Spirn PW, Conant EF, Steiner RM, Needleman L. Thrombosis and infection caused by thoracic venous catheters: pathogenesis and imaging findings. AJR 1993;160:467–471.
21. Smith VC, Hallett JW Jr. Subclavian vein thrombosis during prolonged catheterization for parenteral nutrition: early management and long-term follow-up. Thromb Parent Nutr 1983;76:603–606.
22. Lokich JJ, Becker B. Subclavian vein thrombosis in patients treated with infusion chemotherapy for advanced malignancy. Cancer 1983;52:1586–1589.
23. Brismar B, Hardstedt C, Jacobson S. Diagnosis of thrombosis by catheter phlebography after prolonged central venous catheterization. Ann Surg 11981;94:779–783.
24. Leiby JM, Purcell H, DeMaria JJ, Kraut EH, Sagone AL, Metz EN. Pulmonary embolism as a result of Hickman catheter-related thrombosis. Am J Med 1989;86:228–231.
25. Kaye GC, Smith DR, Johnston D. Fatal right ventricular thrombus secondary to Hickman catheterisation. BJCP 1990;11:780–781.
26. Anderson AJ, Krasnow SH, Boyer MW, et al. Thrombosis: the major Hickman catheter complication in patients with solid tumor. Chest 1989;95:71–75.
27. McDonough JJ, Altemeier WA. Subclavian venous thrombosis secondary to indwelling catheters. Surg Gynecol Obstet 1971;133:397–400.
28. Moss JF, Wagman LD, Riihimaki DU, Terz JJ. Central venous thrombosis related to the silastic Hickman-Broviac catheters in an oncologic population. JPEN 1989;13:397–400.
29. Chastre J, Cornud F, Bouchama A, Biau F, Benacerraf R, Gilbert C. Thrombosis as a complication of pulmonary-artery catheterization via the internal jugular vein. N Engl J Med 1982;3066:278–281.
30. Haire WD, Lieberman RP, Edney J, et al. Hickman catheter-induced thoracic vein thrombosis. Cancer 1990;66:900–908.
31. Jacobson S, Brismar B. Blood hemoglobin: a possible predictor of central venous catheter-related thrombosis in parenteral nutrition. JPEN 1985;9:471–473.

32. Falk RL, Smith DF. Thrombosis of upper extremity thoracic inlet veins: diagnosis with duplex doppler sonography. AJR 1987;149:677–6682.
33. Horner SM, Bell JA, Swanton RH. Infected right atrial thrombus-an important but rare complication of central venous lines. Eur Heart J 1993;14:138–140.
34. Bolz DD, Aadahl P, Mangersnes J, et al. Intravascular ultrasonographic assessment of thrombus formation on central venous catheters. Acta Radiol 1993;34:162–167.
35. Mori H, Fukuda T, Isomoto I, Maeda H, Hayashi K. CT diagnosis of catheter-induced septic thrombus of vena cava. J Comput Assist Tomogr 1990;14:236–238.
36. Kramer FL, Goodman J, Allen S. Thrombolytic therapy in catheter-related subclavian venous thrombosis. J Can Assoc Radiol 1987;38:106–108.
37. Lacey SR, Zartisky AL, Azizkhan RG. Successful treatment of Candida-infected caval thrombosis in critically ill infants by low-dose streptokinase infusion. J Pediatr Surg 1988;23:1204–1209.
38. Lewis JA, LaFrance R, Bower RH. Treatment of an infected silicone right atrial catheter with combined fibrinolytic and antibiotic therapy: case report and review of the literature. JPEN 1989;13:92–98.
39. Fraschini G, Jadeja J, Lawson M, Holmes FA, Carrasco HC, Wallace S. Local infusion of urokinase for the lysis of thrombosis associated with permanent central venous catheters in cancer patients. J Clin Oncol 1987;5:672–678.
40. Rubenstein M, Creger WP. Successful streptokinase therapy for catheter-induced subclavian vein thrombosis. Arch Intern Med 1980;140:1370–1371.
41. Landercasper J, Gall W, Fischer M, et al. Thrombolytic therapy of axillary-subclavian venous thrombosis. Arch Surg 1987;122:1072–1075.
42. Curnow A, Idowu J, Behrens E, Toomey F, Georgeson K. Urokinase therapy for silastic catheter-induced intravascular thrombi in infants and children. Arch Surg 1985;120:1237–1240.
43. Fabri PJ, Mirtallo JM, Ruberg RL, et al. Incidence and prevention of thrombosis of the subclavian vein during total parenteral nutrition. Surg Gynecol Obstet 1982;155:238–240.
44. Brismar B, Hardstedt C, Jacobson S, Kager L, Malmborg A-S. Reduction of catheter-associated thrombosis in parenteral nutrition by intravenous heparin therapy. Arch Surg 1982;117:1196–1199.
45. Hoar PF, Wilson RM, Mangano DT, Avery GJ, Szarnicki RJ, Hill JD. Heparin bonding reduces thrombogenicity of pulmonary-artery catheters. N Engl J Med 1981;305:993–995.
46. Bern MM, Lokich JJ, Wallach SR, et al. Very low doses of warfarin can prevent thrombosis in central venous catheters. Ann Intern Med 1990;112:423–428.

7

Infectious Complications Associated with Long-Term Venous Access Devices: Etiology, Diagnosis, Treatment, and Prophylaxis

H. Richard Alexander

Types of Catheter-Related Infections
Etiology of Catheter-Related Bacteremia
Diagnosis of Catheter-Related Infection
Treatment
Prophylaxis
References

The development of catheter-related septicemia represents the most serious complication of venous access. Early recognition, sensitive and rapid methods of diagnosis, and aggressive treatment are clearly necessary to avoid the potentially life threatening consequences of untreated bacteremia. Because most patients with cancer who have long-term indwelling venous catheters will experience periods of immune compromise secondary to their disease or its treatment, it is not surprising that infectious complications have been reported to range from 3% up to 60%.[1–5]

Types of Catheter-Related Infections

Catheter-related infections can be divided into three types on the basis of clinical grounds. *Exit site* infections originate at the site where an external device exits the skin. These infections are localized processes manifested by erythema and induration around the exit site without systemic signs of infection. The associated tenderness should also be localized to the point of erythema and the subcutaneous tract of the catheter is not involved in the process. In an immunocompromised patient the presence of erythema and exudate may be subtle. Most exit site infections are secondary to *Staphylococcus epidermidis*,[6–9] and initial management with aggressive local wound care and appropriate antibiotics without removing the catheter is indicated and frequently successful.[8,10,11] Patients typically do not appear ill so that this approach appears justified as initial management. The catheter may be used during this period although it is prudent to discontinue chemotherapy until the infection has resolved. If the exit site infection is secondary to a partially extruded Dacron cuff the condition will not respond to local care. In addition, there is a very high risk of the being catheter pulled out inadvertently when the cuff is partially or totally extruded and for these reasons it should be removed under controlled conditions. If, during the course of initial treatment, there is evidence of developing bacteremia associated with an exit site infection, particularly if the isolated pathogen is *Staphylococcus aureus*, catheter removal may be necessary in up to 90% of cases.[12] Most reports on this topic do not define standardized criteria for catheter removal so the conditions under which the catheter should be removed are most appropriately based on clinical judgment.

The second type of infectious complication occurring with external catheters or implanted ports is termed *tunnel* or *pocket* infection and represents a suppurative process through the subcutaneous portion of a catheter (tunnel) or around the implanted port housing. These infections are frequently associated with varying degrees of surrounding cellulitis and systemic signs of infection may be present. The diagnosis is made on clinical grounds with erythema, induration, and tenderness present along the subcutaneous tunnel tract or around the subcutaneous port pocket. The etiology of tunnel or pocket infections is likely to be secondary to the migration of bacteria from the exit site of an external catheter or introduction of bacteria into the port pocket via repeated access with the Huber point needle. Experimental evidence for this phenomenon has been provided by the demonstration that bacteria inoculated at the entry site of subdermally placed 4 cm catheters in laboratory animals can be identified at the tips of the catheters within 1 hour.[13] This migration can occur even when the exit site is swabbed with bacteria 1 week after catheter placement, suggesting that scrupulous exit site care and pocket site asepsis during access of implanted ports are critical to catheter function.

Frequently, purulent fluid can be expressed from the subcutaneous tunnel or aspirated from the port pocket. By virtue of the fact that these infections are suppurative, occur in the presence of a foreign body, and are accompanied by a local cellulitis, it is necessary to remove the catheter or implanted port and use appropriate antibiotics. In addition to removal of the device, adequate drainage of any abscesses or in advanced cases, tissue debridement, is necessary. If Gram stain of purulent fluid does not reveal bacteria then acid-fast staining should be done. Rapidly growing atypical mycobacterial infection of the tunnel or exit site is a rare but virulent type of infection. Flynn et al have reported six cases of rapidly growing atypical *Mycobacterium* spp. as the source of tunnel infections when Gram stain failed to reveal an organism.[14] In these instances catheter removal, antibiotic therapy, and excision of the infected tissue may be necessary to resolve the infection.

Line sepsis or *catheter-related bacteremia* is the most serious and potentially life-threatening infectious complication of chronic indwelling venous catheters and is manifested by clinical signs and symptoms of bacteremia with no other source of infection identified based on clinical and laboratory tests. The etiology, diagnosis, treatment, and prophylaxis of line sepsis are complex issues to which the remainder of this chapter is focused.

Etiology of Catheter-Related Bacteremia

The pathogenesis of catheter-related sepsis appears to be caused primarily by the colonization of the intravascular portion of the catheter by bacteria, most commonly the patient's skin flora, that migrate along the external surface of the catheter from the exit site or are flushed through the lumen from the catheter hubs.[15-17] As mentioned previously, there is experimental evidence that demonstrates the ability of bacteria inoculated at the exit site of a subdermally placed plastic catheter to migrate rapidly and be detected 4 cm from the entry site within 1 hour.[13] Several studies have shown that the most common organism isolated from cultures of catheter tips are skin flora such as *Staphylococcus epidermidis, Staphylococcus aureus,* and *Strep-*

tococcus spp.[18,19] In patients suspected of having catheter-related bacteremia, there is a strong correlation between isolates obtained from external sites on a catheter and the catheter tip.[18]

Once bacteria gain access to the intravascular portion of the catheter, colonization may be facilitated by the presence of a biofilm which is typically present on long-term venous access catheters. By means of electron microscopy, bacterial colonization of Gram positive cocci has been observed in an adherent glycocalyx biofilm present on 13 of 15 (87%) long-term venous catheter lumens in cancer patients.[15] Of note, a confluent biofilm was present on some portion of all catheters examined that were in place for greater than 3 months. The presence of thrombus on central venous catheters has also correlated strongly with bacterial colonization.[17] Cooper and Hopkins have reported that direct Gram stain of various types of catheters removed for suspicion of infection correlated with the subsequent confirmation of catheter colonization established by positive catheter tip cultures (15 colonies per blood agar plate).[16] Direct Gram staining of the catheter tips revealed adherent microorganisms and was 100% sensitive and 96.9% specific for the detection of catheter tip colonization. Although direct Gram staining was proposed as a rapid diagnostic method for catheter-associated infection, this technique is clearly not appropriate for routine use because most patients can be treated successfully for catheter-related infection while the catheter remains in situ. These observations do support, however, the concept that organisms originating at external catheter sites migrate to and reside in the glycocalyx biofilm adherent to long-term venous access catheters and may provide a source of catheter-related bacteremia. The generally lower rates of infectious complications in patients with subcutaneously implanted ports may be a reflection of the fact that when the port is not in use there is no communication between the skin flora and the catheter. However, in cases of implanted port related bacteremia the etiology may be similar to that of external catheters in that skin flora introduced into the port pocket or housing via the access needle may migrate and colonize the catheter.

The importance of neutropenia as a contributing factor to the development of catheter related infection has been addressed by several studies primarily in pediatric cancer patients. In children undergoing treatment for cancer, van Hoff et al have reported a retrospective cohort study in which there was a six fold increase in sepsis rates and more time spent in the hospital when long-term venous access catheters were used compared to intermittent peripheral venous access catheters.[20] With a multivariate analysis to control for disease status, intensity of chemotherapy, diagnosis, age, sex, and the presence of a venous access catheter, the relative risk of developing sepsis was highest in children with catheters and in those with more advanced disease. The development of fever and neutropenia was only marginally affected by the presence of a catheter (relative risk: 1.56, $P = .053$). Similarly, Gorelick et al have shown that the incidence of

TABLE 7-1
Incidence and Types of Infection in Pediatric Patients with Long-Term Venous Access Catheters with and Without Neutropenia

Type of Infection	Neutropenic (N = 85)	Non-neutropenic (N = 55)
Bacteremia	8 (9)*	13 (24)†
Exit site infection	12 (14)	15 (27)
Combined	0 (0)	9 (16)‡
Total catheter-related infection	20 (24)	19 (35)

*Numbers in parentheses, percent.
†$P<.05$.
‡$P<.01$.
From Gorelick MH, Owen WC, Seibel NL, Reaman GH. Lack of association between neutropenia and the incidence of bacteremia associated with indwelling central venous catheters in febrile pediatric cancer patients. Pediatr Infect Dis J 1991;10:506–510. Used with permission.

bacteremia in pediatric cancer patients with long-term venous access catheters is not higher in the presence of neutropenia.[21] In 67 patients there were 140 episodes of fever of which 39% developed in patients without neutropenia and 61% occurred during periods with neutropenia. There was a higher association of bacteremia in patients without neutropenia, but the infection rates were comparable when clinical evidence of an exit site infection was absent (Table 7-1). The most common bacterial isolates in both groups were Gram-Positive organisms-*Staphylococcus aureus* and coagulase-negative staphylococci. Polymicrobial infections were rare. Viscoli et al have also reported on the lack of an association between the rates of catheter-related infections and the presence of neutropenia (<1000 neutrophils/mm^3) in children with cancer.[5,22] Although 88% of catheter-unrelated infections and 96% of infections of unknown origin developed during periods of neutropenia, only 48% of catheter-related infections occurred during neutropenia. In catheter-related infections, Gram-positive organisms accounted for 78% of all isolates, of which half were staphylococci.

These data indicate that the incidence of bacteremia during a febrile episode in cancer patients is comparable in patients with or without neutropenia. The incidence of bacteremia during febrile episodes appears high enough (10%) to justify the use of prophylactic antibiotics in this setting.

Diagnosis of Catheter-Related Infection

A rapid and reliable method of diagnosing catheter-related bacteremia while the catheter remains in situ would be ideal and a number of studies have addressed this issue. Initially, other sources of infection based on clinical and laboratory findings should be excluded. The utility of a semiquantitative culture technique in diagnosing catheter-related infections has been described by Maki et al.[23] Their work has demonstrated that when more than 15 colonies grew from a vascular access catheter tip on a blood agar plate culture, the likelihood of having an associated catheter-related septicemia was significantly greater than with a count of fewer than 15 colonies per plate. Of note, when the semiquantitative culture technique was used on catheters from patients experiencing bacteremia from documented other remote sites, no concordant isolates were identified. Therefore this technique appears to be a very sensitive method of distinguishing catheter-related infection from other sites of infection.

Andremont et al have evaluated the utility of semiquantitative blood cultures drawn through the catheter to predict the probability of catheter tip colonization in cancer patients.[18] Semiquantitative cultures were obtained from the tips and hubs of more than 200 long-term venous access catheters in cancer patients. Overall, cultures were positive from 18% of the hub and 29% of the tip cultures. When more than 1000 colony-forming units per ml (CFU/mL) were obtained from the hub culture the probability of a positive catheter tip culture of the same organism (15 CFU/mL) was almost 90% (Table 7-2). However, if fewer than 1000 CFU/mL were obtained from the catheter hub the predictive value fell markedly. Interestingly, there were 30 positive tip cultures in which external hub cultures were negative. The most common isolates were *Staphyloccus epidermidis* and *Staphyloccus aureus*. Cercenado et al have also studied the value of exit site and hub cultures in diagnosing catheter-associated infection.[19] Of 139 cathe-

TABLE 7-2
Comparison Between the Results of 205 Paired Cultures of Hub Blood and Central Venous Catheter Tips in Adult Cancer Patients

Microbial Concentration in Hub Blood Culture (CFU/mL)	No. of Hub Blood Cultures	No. of Catheter Tips Colonized*	Likelihood Ratio†
>1000	11	10	31.0
101–1000	6	3	3.1
1–100	21	21	1.6
0	167	30‡	0.7

*Colonization was arbitrarily defined as a catheter tip culture containing more than 15 CFUs of the same organism as observed in the corresponding hub blood culture.
†Likelihood ratios were calculated for each different microbial concentration.
‡Presence of more than 15 CFU in the catheter tip culture (all species).
From Adremont A, Paulet R, Nitenberg G, Hill C. Value of semiquantitative cultures of blood drawn through catheter hubs for estimating the risk of catheter tip colonization in cancer patients. J Clin Microbiol 1988;26:2297–2299. Used with permission.

ters, both peripheral cannulae and central, 53 catheters were identified as infected based on semiquantitative culture (15 CFU plate). All but three of these had positive cultures of identical microorganisms isolated from either the exit site, the hub, or both sites. In 79 cases accompanied by clinical suspicion of infection, 34 of 35 had both tip and superficial (hub or exit site) positive cultures. In the 60 remaining cases where there was no clinical suspicion of infection, 11 of 18 had both tip and hub positive cultures. Of note, all catheters with negative superficial cultures had a negative tip culture. In contrast to the study by Andremont et al,[18] these data suggest that when negative superficial cultures are obtained, even in the presence of a clinical suspicion of catheter-related infection, the diagnosis of catheter-associated infection appeared unlikely. When superficial cultures produce more than 1000 CFU/mL the likelihood of a positive tip culture is 90%.

Because most patients can be treated successfully for catheter-related bacteremia with the catheter in situ other methods of diagnosing catheter related bacteremia have been described. Wing et al described a patient with suspected catheter-related bacteremia in whom quantitative cultures from peripheral blood and blood drawn through the catheter were compared.[24] In this case report, the catheter was removed on the basis of an enormous (>400-fold) difference in the number of colonies per milliliter obtained from peripheral blood and catheter blood cultures. Catheter-related sepsis was subsequently confirmed by catheter tip culture.

The experimental evidence that supports the utility of a greater than fivefold increase in colony count in blood sampled through the catheter vs peripheral blood cultures for diagnosing catheter-related bacteremia has been established by Flynn and co-workers.[25] They produced bacteremia by inoculating *Escherichia coli* intraperitoneally into rabbits with indwelling central and peripheral (femoral) venous lines. During the subsequent 3 1/2 hours after the bacterial challenge a septicemia developed and quantitative blood cultures were obtained simultaneously from both venous lines at various intervals. The concentration of bacteria was significantly greater in the superior vena cava than in femoral blood with a mean ratio of 2.2. The mean superior vena cava/femoral vein ratio plus three standard deviations of the mean was 4.34 (which included 99% of all bacteremias). These data indicate that a ratio of CFUs of five-fold or less is compatible with a bacteremia from a remote site while a greater than five-fold difference may be considered indicative of catheter-related bacteremia.

In children with suspected catheter-related bacteremia, Raucher et al have also shown that a comparison of quantitative blood cultures drawn from the catheter and peripheral vein is a rapid and accurate method of diagnosing catheter-related infection.[26] Quantitative and nonquantitative (broth) cultures were obtained from 14 children during 30 febrile episodes and were sterile in 19. In two other children broth cultures identified identical organisms and a remote source of infection was found in both. In the remaining nine children, quantita-

TABLE 7-3
Criteria for the Diagnosis of Catheter-Related Bacteremia

Clinical signs of infection; no other source identified
Positive blood cultures from the catheter show a five- to tenfold (or greater) colony count vs peripheral cultures
Greater than 100 CFU/mL from catheter
Temporal relationship between catheter manipulation and development of symptoms

tive cultures from the catheter became positive within 16 hours; six of these had counts greater than 2000 CFU/mL. In five of six children in whom simultaneous peripheral quantitative cultures were obtained less than 30 CFU/ml were identified. In this study as well as others,[27] the routine use of surveillance cultures to predict impending line-related sepsis was not helpful.

Based on available information the following criteria appear to be sufficient for diagnosing catheter-related infections: (1) clinical signs of infection without evidence of a remote source, (2) semiquantitative or quantitative positive blood cultures collected through the catheter show a five to tenfold or greater colony count compared to peripheral blood cultures or, (3) an absolute count of 100 CFU/mL or greater from the indwelling venous catheter is identified alone.[11,25] In addition, if there is a relationship between the timing of catheter care, that is, flushing, and the development of symptoms of bacteremia (ie, fever and chills) there should be suspicion that manipulation of the catheter may have precipitated the episode (Table 7-3).

Treatment

A number of studies have reported successful treatment of line sepsis while the catheter remains in situ.[3,11,22,25,28,29] In a series of 88 episodes of culture-proven catheter-related bacteremia in adults with long-term venous access catheters, Benezra et al[11] have shown that treatment was successful in 33 of 54 patients (61%) with antibiotics alone. Successful treatment of line sepsis was defined as negative culture results after a course of antibiotics and failure was defined as persistently positive culture results after antibiotic therapy or the development of recurrent infections with the same organism. The time to onset of line-related sepsis was extremely variable, ranging from 5 to 335 days after insertion. The isolates obtained were predominately Gram-positive in those successfully treated with antibiotics alone (Table 7-4).

Two studies in children with venous catheters have used comparative semiquantitative blood cultures taken from the catheter and a peripheral site to diagnose catheter-related bacteremia.[22,25] The criteria for a diagnosis of catheter-related bacteremia in these studies were either positive blood cultures taken through the catheter with sterile

TABLE 7-4

Outcome of Antibiotic Therapy in Catheter-Related Sepsis is Dependent on Microorganism

Organism	Cured (N = 33)	Failed (N = 21)
Coagulase-negative staphylococci	8	2
Staphylococcus aureus	3	0
Bacillus spp.	1	2
Streptococcus faecalis	0	2
Enterobacteriaceae	5	2
Pseudomonas spp.	4	4
Acinetobacter spp.	2	1
Candida spp.	1	0
Polymicrobic	9	8

From Benezra D, Kiehn TE, Gold JWM, Brown AE, Turnbull ADM, Armstrong D. Prospective study of infections in indwelling central venous catheters using quantitative blood cultures. Am J Med 1988;85:495–498. Used with permission.

peripheral cultures or a greater than fivefold concentration of bacteria in catheter blood compared to peripheral blood. Viscoli et al[22] reported that antibiotic therapy with catheters in situ was successful in 12 of 21 patients (57%). In this study half of the catheter-related bacteremias occurred in children with neutropenia. Although it is not stated, one could presume that a similar proportion of neutropenic children were successfully treated with antibiotics alone. Four of the nine line related bacteremias that were not successfully treated were noted to have associated tunnel infections. It is reasonable to expect that in patients with line-related sepsis and without any local signs of infection, the likelihood of successful treatment with antibiotics alone even in the presence of neutropenia is high. Flynn et al[25] have similarly reported that antibiotic treatment alone administered through the catheter was successful in eradicating line-related bacteremia in 11 of 17 children with cancer.

Hartman and Shochat reported the successful treatment of line-related septicemia in 25 of 28 children (89%) including Gram-negative, Gram-positive, multiple-organism septicemia in four patients, and candida fungemia in three.[3] Catheter-related bacteremia was defined as a positive blood culture obtained from the central venous catheter in the presence of fever and no localizing signs. However, the fact that only 30% of patients had additional peripheral blood cultures may indicate that some of these septic episodes were not actually secondary to line sepsis. Nonneutropenic patients were treated with parenteral antibiotics for 10 to 14 days and negative follow-up cultures were obtained after cessation of therapy.

A major question in the treatment of catheter-related bacteremia is: Under what conditions should the infected catheter be removed? Clearly, a deteriorating clinical condition while the patient is on appropriate antibiotics should be treated with urgent catheter removal. Recurrent infections and persistently positive blood cultures after completion of treatment are other indications for catheter removal. The rate of *Candida* spp. infections in patients with long-term venous access are twice as common in infants and children than in adults (3.8% vs 1.2%, respectively) and complications secondary to fungemia appear to more severe in the younger age group.[30] Eppes et al reviewed the outcomes of infants with predominantly noncancer diagnoses who had various types of central venous or arterial catheters and were treated with amphotericin B for *Candida* spp. fungemia.[31] Infants treated with the catheter in situ had higher rates of persistent fungemia and adverse outcomes compared to those whose catheters were removed (Table 7-5). In children with long term venous access catheters and catheter-related candida fungemia, Dato and Dajani found that patients fared better when catheters were removed.[30] Four of five deaths occurred in patients whose catheters remained in place for 5 days or longer after blood cultures, were obtained. On the other hand, Hartman and Shochat[3] noted that three of four children with catheter-related fungemia were successfully treated with the catheter insitu. However, in eight patients with fungal or multiple organism sepsis, the only death occurred in a 13-year-old patient with an unspecified fungemia.

Dugdale and Ramsey have presented evidence that catheter-related *Staphylococcus aureus* infections in adults with long-term venous access catheters appear to carry a worse prognosis and to have a lower likelihood of successful in situ therapy than other bacterial catheter related infections.[12] Among 41 episodes of bacteremia only eight were cured without catheter removal. However, among the 41

TABLE 7-5

Microbiologic and Clinical Outcomes for Candidemia Associated with Central Venous or Arterial Catheters Treated with Amphotericin B

	Catheter Removed (N = 13)	Catheter Retained (N = 8)	P-Values
No. with persistent candidemia	2	6	.018 (Fisher's exact test)
Median duration of candidemia	0 day	4 days	.004 (Kruskal–Wallis test)
Morbidity (subsequent complications of candidemia)	2	3	NS
Candida-related death	0	2	.13 (Fisher's exact test)
Adverse outcome (subsequent morbidity, mortality, persistent candidemia)	3	7	.008 (Fisher's exact test)
Failure of catheter within 14 days of intervention (continued fungemia, bacteremia, malfunction)		7/8	

NS, not significant
From Eppes SC, Troutman JL, Gutman LT. Outcome of treatment of candidemia in children whose central catheters were removed or retained. Pediatr Infect Dis 1989;8:99–104. Used with permission.

cases were 15 with coexistent tunnel or exit site infections. Even if all eight patients cured were among the other 26 patients, the cure rate without catheter removal would be only 31%, substantially less than the percentage reported for other bacterial infections in other series. Almost all patients with signs of exit site or tunnel infection required catheter removal for cure.

Fifteen cases of *Mycobacterium fortuitum* complex infection in cancer patients with long-term venous access catheters have been described by Raad.[32] All seven patients in whom the catheter was retained and who were treated with antibiotics alone suffered treatment failure whereas the other four patients treated with catheter removal and antibiotics recovered. *Bacillus* spp. infections have also been reported to be resistant to in-situ treatment.[33] Therefore, although most cases of catheter-related bacteremias can be successfully treated in situ with systemic antibiotics, certain pathogens such as *Staphylococcus aureus*, *Candida* spp., *Mycobacterium* spp., and *Bacillus* spp. are more difficult to eradicate and early catheter removal should be considered seriously. In all patients with catheter-related infection the decision to remove the catheter should be based on the close clinical assessment of the patient and response to initial antibiotic therapy. If there is persistent evidence of infection or any deterioration in the condition of the patient, the catheter should be removed.

Prophylaxis

Several prospective randomized trials have evaluated the efficacy of a silver ion impregnated catheter cuff (VitaCuff, Vitaphore, CA) that is placed subcutaneously around a central venous catheter and designed to prevent catheter colonization from exit site flora.[34-37] The duration of the antimicrobial effect of the silver-impregnated cuff is approximately 6 weeks and presumably any clinical effect should be observed during this time period. Three studies have evaluated its effectiveness in percutaneously placed central venous catheters.[34,35] Maki et al[35] reported the results of a multicenter trial in which over 200 temporary central venous catheters were inserted with or without the cuff in hospitalized patients for a wide variety of indications including hyperalimentation, hemodialysis, or pulmonary artery catheterization prior to open heart surgery. Results showed that catheters inserted with the cuff had a significantly lower rate of local catheter-related infection (15 CFU) than catheters placed without the cuff (9% vs 29%). Although the incidence of catheter-related bacteremias was also lower in the cuff group (1% vs 3.7%), the overall number of catheter related bacteremias in the study was low so that the difference was not statistically significantly different (Table 7-6). Of interest, the cuff was not effective in reducing catheter-related infection when the catheter was used to replace an existing catheter over a guidewire (Table 7-6). In a second randomized control trial in which

TABLE 7-6
Catheter-Related Infections in Temporary Central Venous Catheters Inserted with or Without a Silver Ion Impregnated Cuff

| Type of | Type of Catheter | |
Catheter-Related Infection	Controls	Cuffed
Newly inserted (total N)	135	99
Local*	33 (28.9%)	7 (9.1%)
Bacteremia	5 (3.7%)	1 (10%)
Replaced over guidewire (total N)	59	51
Local	7 (12%)	8 (16%)
Bacteremia	2 (3%)	1 (2%)

*$P = .002$.
Modified from Maki DG, Cobb L, Garman JK, Shapiro JM, Ringer M, Helgerson RB. An attachable silver-impregnated cuff for prevention of infection with central venous catheters: a prospective randomized multicenter trial. Am J Med 1988;85:307–314.

temporary central venous catheters with or without cuffs were inserted in surgical intensive care unit patients, Flowers et al have reported similar results.[34] Twenty-six cuffed and 29 uncuffed catheters were inserted after randomization. The rate of colonization was significantly higher in the uncuffed catheter group (34.5% vs 7.7%). Similar to the study reported byaki, the incidence of catheter-related bacteremia was higher in the control group (13.8% vs 0%) but the number of bacteremias overall was too small to show a statistically significant difference between the groups. Of interest in this study, a large proportion of catheter-related infections were due to *Candida albicans* which may have been due to the use of polyantibiotic ointment.

Bonawitz et al[37] have reported the results of a four arm prospective randomized trial in which patients admitted to a surgical intensive care unit and who required a central venous catheter were assigned to receive or not receive a cuffed catheter and to have the catheter removed either 3 or 7 days after insertion. When grouped according to the use of a silver-impregnated cuff the colonization rates were similar with or without the cuff (14.5% vs 18.1%) as were the rates of infection (5.3% vs 0%, respectively). Of note, there was a high dropout rate in this study (20%) from either accidental catheter removal, death of the patient, or failure to obtain cultures.

Recently, a prospective randomized trial has been completed evaluating the effect of the silver-impregnated cuff in tunneled long term vascular access catheters in cancer patients.[36] More than 200 patients with various malignancies were randomly assigned to receive a standard dual-lumen 10 French Leonard catheter with or without a silver-impregnated cuff. There was no difference in any parameter between groups including the number of local or systemic infectious complications or the indications for catheter removal. The results of this study provide some indirect information about the relative importance of catheter colonization from bacterial migration from the exit site along the subcutaneous tunnel of the catheter. The rate of tunnel or local infection in this study was extremely low (1%) and attests to the importance and effectiveness of patient teaching in home maintenance exit site protocols. The silver-impregnated cuff will not affect the colonization of bacteria from the catheter hubs. With the use of scrupulous exit site care there does not appear to be any additional benefit from the addition of a silver-impregnated cuff in this setting. Furthermore, if the majority of catheter-related bacteremias in this study were primarily from colonization of bacteria from the hub, further studies to define the optimal flushing routine to minimize catheter contamination while maintaining patency are needed.

Schwartz et al have reported the results of a prospective randomized trial evaluating the utility of an antibiotic flush vs heparin alone in reducing luminal colonization of long-term venous access catheters in pediatric oncology patients.[38] Previous work has shown that heparin does not have any antimicrobial activity against *Staphylococcusepidermidis*, a common catheter isolate.[39] In this study, children were randomly assigned to receive either 10 U/mL of heparin alone or 10 U/mL of heparin with 25 µg/mL of vancomycin for all catheter flushes. There was a significantly lower number of catheter-related bacteremias and a significantly longer infection-free interval from vancomycin-sensitive organisms when the antibiotic flush was used. There were five bacteremias due to coagulase-negative *Staphylococcus* spp. in the heparin flush group compared with none in the antibiotic flush group. Not surprisingly, there was no difference in the number of infections due to vancomycin-resistant organisms or exit site infections. Peripheral levels of vancomycin could not be detected with the doses administered through the catheter and the emergence of antibiotic-resistant isolates was not observed.

If colonization occurs to any substantial degree during the time of catheter insertion then short-term prophylactic antibiotics might be effective in reducing catheter-related infections. Two randomized prospective studies have produced conflicting results. Ranson et al have reported the results of a double-blind prospective randomized trial of perioperative vancomycin vs placebo in adult cancer patients undergoing long-term venous access catheter insertion.[40] Patients were stratified according to diagnosis and severity of treatment. Treatment with either vancomycin, 500 mg, or placebo was instituted just prior to catheter insertion and a second dose was administered 20 to 30 minutes after satisfactory insertion of the catheter had been completed. For leukemia patients undergoing bone marrow transplantation there was an overall rate of 57% of catheter-related bacteremia of which coagulase-negative staphylococcus was the most common isolate. There was no difference in the rate of catheter-related bacteremia in vancomycin- or placebo-treated groups in the first 30 days or during the entire catheter life. For patients with solid tumors the total incidence of catheter-related bacteremia was lower than that for the previous group. Similarly, there was no difference in catheter-related bacteremias with or without antibiotic treatment. In a second study, Lim et al evaluated the effectiveness of single-dose teicoplanin, a long-acting antibiotic structurally related to vancomycin.[41] Eighty-eight cancer patients undergoing placement of long-term venous access catheters were randomized to receive a single 400-mg dose of intravenous teicoplanin 2 to 4 hours prior to catheter insertion. Patient characteristics were evenly distributed between groups with respect to the usual pertinent clinical criteria. Local infectious complications (exit site, tunnel infection) occurred with equal frequency between groups. In patients receiving prophylactic teicoplanin there was a significantly lower incidence of early catheter-related Gram-positive bacteremia (17.5% vs 40%). The total number of Gram-positive isolates was also lower in the antibiotic-treated group whereas the number of Gram-negative organisms isolated was not different. These data would seem to support the use of prophylactic antibiotic use in patients undergoing intensive chemotherapy with probable neutropenia. A confirmatory trial with a larger cohort and including patients with less intensive treatment schedules will be necessary prior to the routine use of perioperative antibiotics during the insertion of long-term venous access catheters.

References

1. Shaw JHF, Douglas R, Wilson T. Clinical performance of Hickman and Port-A-Cath atrial catheters. Aust N Z J Surg 1988;58:657–659.
2. Greene FL, Moore W, Strickland G, McFarland J. Comparison of a totally implantable access device for chemotherapy (Port-A-Cath) and long-term percutaneous catheterization (Broviac). South Med J 1988;81:580–603.
3. Hartman GE, Shochat SJ. Management of septic complications associated with Silastic catheters in childhood malignancy. Pediatr Infect Dis J 1987;6:1042–1047.
4. Hiemenz J, Skelton J, Pizzo PA. Perspective on the management of catheter-related infections in cancer patients. Pediatr Infect Dis J 1986;5:6–11.
5. Viscoli C. Aspects of infections in children with cancer. Recent Results Cancer Res 1988;108:71–81.
6. Press OW, Ramsey PG, Larson EB, Fefer A, Hickman RO. Hickman catheter infections in patients with malignancies. Medicine 1984;63:189–200.
7. Krog MPM, Ekborn A, Nystrom-Rosander C, Rudberg CR, Simonsson NOB. Central venous catheters in acute blood malignancies. Cancer 1987;59:1358–1361.
8. Harvey MP, Trent RJ, Joshua DE, Ramsey-Stewart G, Storey DW, Kronenberg H. Complications associated with indwelling venous

Hickman catheters in patients with hematological disorders. Aust N Z J Med 1986;16:211–215.
9. Schuman ES, Winters V, Gross GF, Hayes JF. Management of Hickman catheter sepsis. Am J Surg 1985;149:627–628.
10. Raaf JH. Results from use of 826 vascular access devices in cancer patients. Cancer 1985;55:1312–1321.
11. Benezra D, Kiehn TE, Gold JWM, Brown AE, Turnbull ADM, Armstrong D. Prospective study of infections in indwelling central venous catheters using quantitative blood cultures. Am J Med 1988;85:495–498.
12. Dugdale DC, Ramsey PG. *Staphylococcus aureus* bacteremia in patients with Hickman catheters. Am J Med 1990;89:137–141.
13. Cooper GL, Schiller AL, Hopkins CC. Possible role of capillary action in pathogenesis of experimental catheter-associated dermal tunnel infections. J Clin Microbiol 1988;26:8–12.
14. Flynn PM, van Hooser B, Gigliotti F. Atypical mycobacterial infections of Hickman catheter exit sites. Pediatr Infect Dis J 1991; 1988:510–513.
15. Tenney JH, Moody MR, Newman KA, et al. Adherent microorganisms on lumenal surfaces of long-term intravenous catheters. Arch Intern Med 1986;146:1949–1954.
16. Cooper GL, Hopkins CC. Rapid diagnosis of intravascular catheter-associated infection by direct gram staining of catheter segments. N Engl J Med 1985;312:1142–1147.
17. Stillman RM, Soliman F, Garcia L, Sawyer PN. Etiology of catheter-associated sepsis. Arch Surg 1977;112:1497–1499.
18. Andremont A, Paulet R, Nitenberg G, Hill C. Value of semiquantitative cultures of blood drawn through catheter hubs for estimating the risk of catheter tip colonization in cancer patients. J Clin Microbiol 1988;26:2297–2299.
19. Cercenado E, Ena J, Rodriguez-Creixems M, Romero I, Bouza E. A conservative procedure for the diagnosis of catheter-related infections. Arch Intern Med 1990;150:1417–1420.
20. van Hoff J, Berg AT, Seashore JH. The effect of right atrial catheters on infectious complications of chemotherapy in children. J Clin Oncol 1990;8:1255–1262.
21. Gorelick MH, Owen WC, Seibel NL, Reaman GH. Lack of association between neutropenia and the incidence of bacteremia associated with indwelling central venous catheters in febrile pediatric cancer patients. Pediatr Infect Dis J 1991;10:506–510.
22. Viscoli C, Garaventa A, Boni L, et al. Role of Broviac catheters in infections in children with cancer. Pediatr Infect Dis J 1988;7:556–560.
23. Maki DG, Weise CE, Sarafin HW. A semiquantitative culture method for identifying intravenous catheter-related infection. N Engl J Med 1977;296:1305–1309.
24. Wing EJ, Norden CW, Shadduck RK, Winkelstein A. Use of quantitative bacteriologic techniques to diagnose catheter-related sepsis. Arch Intern Med 1979;139:482–483.

25. Flynn PM, Shenep JL, Stokes DC, Barrett FF. *In situ* management of confirmed central venous catheter-related bacteremia. Pediatr Infect Dis J 1987;6:729–734.
26. Raucher HS, Hyatt AC, Barzilai A, et al. Quantitative blood cultures in the evaluation of septicemia in children with Broviac catheters. J Pediatr 1984;104:29–33.
27. Rotstein C, Higby D, Killion K, Powell E. Relationship of surveillance cultures to bacteremia and fungemia in bone marrow transplant recipients with Hickman or broviac catheters. J Surg Oncol 1988;39:154–158.
28. Brar KA, Murray DL, Leader I. Central venous catheter infections in pediatric patients—in a community hospital. Infection 1988;16:86–90.
29. Kappers-Klunne MC, Degener JE, Stijnen T, Abels J. Complications from long-term indwelling central venous catheters in hematologic patients with special reference to infection. Cancer 1989;64:1747–1752.
30. Dato VM, Dajani AS. Candidemia in children with central venous catheters: role of catheter removal and amphotericin B therapy. Pediatr Infect Dis J 1990;9:309–314.
31. Eppes SC, Troutman JL, Gutman LT. Outcome of treatment of candidemia in children whose central catheters were removed or retained. Pediatr Infect Dis J 1989;8:99–104.
32. Raad II, Vartivarian S, Khan A, Bodey GP. Catheter-related infections caused by the *Mycobacterium fortuitum* complex: 15 cases and review. Rev Infect Dis 1991;13:1120–1125.
33. Banerjee C, Bustamante CI, Wharton R, Talley E, Wade JC. Bacillus infections in patients with cancer. Arch Intern Med 1988;148:1769–1774.
34. Flowers RH, III, Schwenzer KJ, Kopel RF, Fisch MJ, Tucker SI, Farr BM. Efficacy of an attachable subcutaneous cuff for the prevention of intravascular catheter-related infection. A randomized controlled trial. JAMA 1989;261:878–883.
35. Maki DG, Cobb L, Garman JK, Shapiro JM, Ringer M, Helgerson RB. An attachable silver-impregnated cuff for prevention of infection with central venous catheters: a prospecive randomized multicenter trial. Am J Med 1988;85:307–314.
36. Groeger JS, Lucas AB, Coit D, et al. A prospective randomized evaluation of the effect of silver impregnated subcutaneous cuffs for preventing tunneled chronic venous access catheter infections in cancer patients. Ann Surg 1993;218:206–210.
37. Bonawitz SC, Hammell EJ, Kirkpatrick JR. Prevention of central venous catheter sepsis: a prospective randomized trial. Am Surg 1991;57:618–623.
38. Schwartz C, Henrickson KJ, Roghmann K, Powell K. Prevention of bacteremia attributed to luminal colonization of tunneled central venous catheters with vancomycin-susceptible organisms. J Clin Oncol 1990;8:1591–1597.
39. Root JL, McIntyre OR, Jacobs NJ, Daghlian CP. Inhibitory effect of

disodium EDTA upon the growth of *Staphylococcus epidermidis in vitro*: relation to infection prophylaxis of Hickman catheters. Antimicrob Agents Chemother 1988;32:1627–1631.
40. Ranson MR, Oppenheim BA, Jackson A, Kamthan AG, Scarffe JH. Double-blind placebo controlled study of vancomycin prophylaxis for central venous catheter insertion in cancer patients. J Hosp Infect 1990;15:95–102.
41. Lim SH, Smith MP, Salooja N, Machin SJ, Goldstone AH. A prospective randomized study of prophylactic teicoplanin to prevent early Hickman catheter-related sepsis in patients receiving intensive chemotherapy for haematological malignancies. J Antimicrob Chemother 1991;28:109–116.

8
New Technologies in Long-Term Venous Access and Peripherally Inserted Central Venous Access Catheters

H. Richard Alexander
Alice B. Lucas

General Features of PICCs
Types of PICCs
Catheter Tracking Devices
Technique of Insertion
Clinical Performance of PICCs
Clinical Performance of Peripherally Implanted Ports
References

Peripherally inserted central catheters (PICCs) are silastic or polyurethane catheters inserted into an antecubital vein and positioned so that the tip resides in the superior vena cava. In the past, peripherally inserted central venous catheters were used for short-term venous access in hospitalized patients. However, the development of stronger and less thrombogenic catheter materials has created a new enthusiasm for PICCs as an alternative method of intermediate to long-term venous access. Although the indications for use is evolving, currently it is thought that antecubital devices may fill an interim need between peripheral access and the placement of a long-term central venous device. Indications for a PICC line may include patients with infectious disease processes in whom long-term antibiotic therapy is required, patients with malignant chest wall involvement, radiation therapy fibrosis, presence of a tracheostomy, open wounds on the upper chest, radical neck dissection, or patients physically unable to undergo a surgical procedure. Patients should also be evaluated on the basis of their ability to participate in their own care because these devices require home maintenance procedures similar to those required for the right atrial silastic catheters.

Some of the advantages associated with the use of these lines include accommodation of treatment that cannot be given through small peripheral veins related to irritation; decreased cost associated with the insertion procedure compared to long-term devices; and fewer potential complications which are usually less severe than with conventionally placed central lines.[1] Several features of PICCs may make them the preferred route of access for some patients and growing experience has been reported that establishes them as a safe and functional source of venous access.

General Features of PICCs

PICCs are available in a variety of French sizes and lengths. The devices may differ in catheter material or in the insertion hardware that accompanies the catheter. Many PICCs are made of polyurethane because it possesses a higher burst pressure and greater shear resistance than silastic materials. In general, PICCs have a smaller diameter and are stiffer than centrally inserted silastic vascular access catheters so that they can be advanced through a peripheral forearm vein, typically the cephalic or basilic vein. They are most commonly used as single lumen external catheters but there are double lumen catheters and single lumen peripheral implanted ports available as well. Although some peripherally inserted venous access devices are designed so that the tip resides in a more peripheral position (so called midline catheters), for the purposes of this chapter, PICCs refer to lines designed to be advanced to the superior vena cava. Because of this position in the high blood flow system of the superior vena cava, the catheter can be used to infuse hyperosmolar solutions such as total parenteral nutrition (TPN) or vesicant or irritating (chemotherapy) solutions. As with other venous access devices, PICCs require routine daily heparin flushes and regular dressing changes. However, the greatest advantages of PICCs are that they can be inserted in an office, bedside, or home setting by specially trained nurses using sterile technique and, compared with centrally inserted vascular access devices, the possibility of inadvertent arterial puncture or pneumothorax is eliminated. Repeated prior venipunctures of the antecubital veins may have produced sufficient injury to preclude their use for PICC insertion. In patients with an indwelling PICC blood pressure should be measured in the contralateral arm to avoid damage to or occlusion of the catheter.

Types of PICCs

PICCs come in a variety of sizes for pediatric or neonatal use ranging from 1.2- to 2.6-French (Fr) and require an introducer needle between 24- and 19-gauge for insertion. The adult catheters range in size from 2.6- to 5.0-Fr and use a 19- to 14-gauge needle for insertion. The adult PICC is typically 50 to 60 cm long and has interval length markings at 5-cm increments for reference (Figure 8-1). A dual-lumen catheter is also available (Figure 8-2). The lumens are configured in an asymmetric "double-D" with one lumen slightly larger than the other (Figure 8-3). The external access hubs on the dual-lumen PICC are staggered in length so that each lumen can be distinguished.

The most recently developed venous access device, the periph-

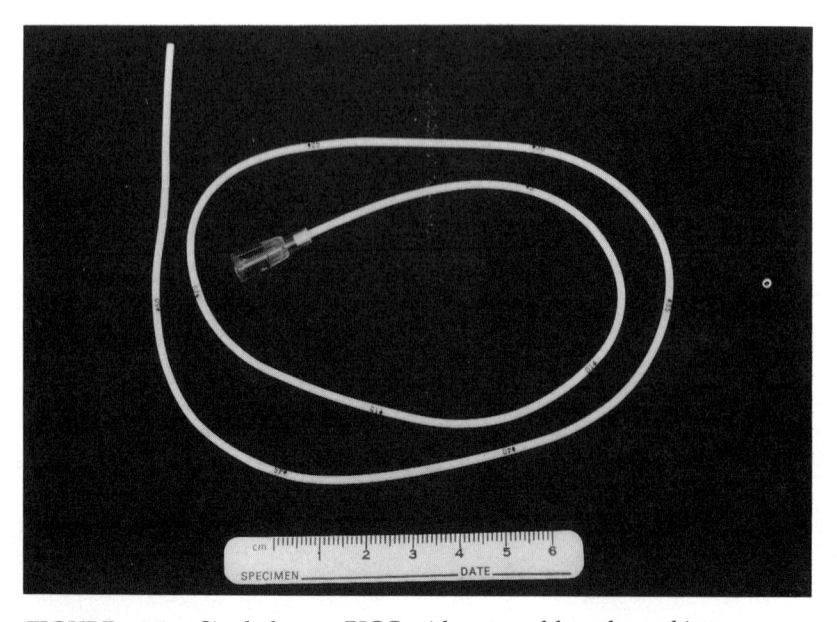

FIGURE 8-1. Single-lumen PICC with external length markings.

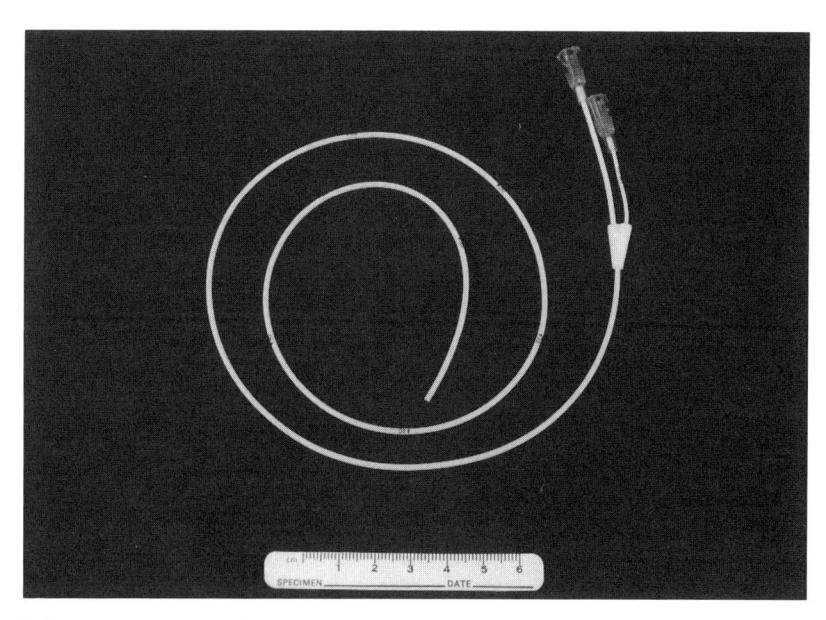

FIGURE 8-2. Double-lumen PICC with external length markings and staggered external hubs so that lumens can be distinguished. The shorter external hub accesses the smaller of the two lumens.

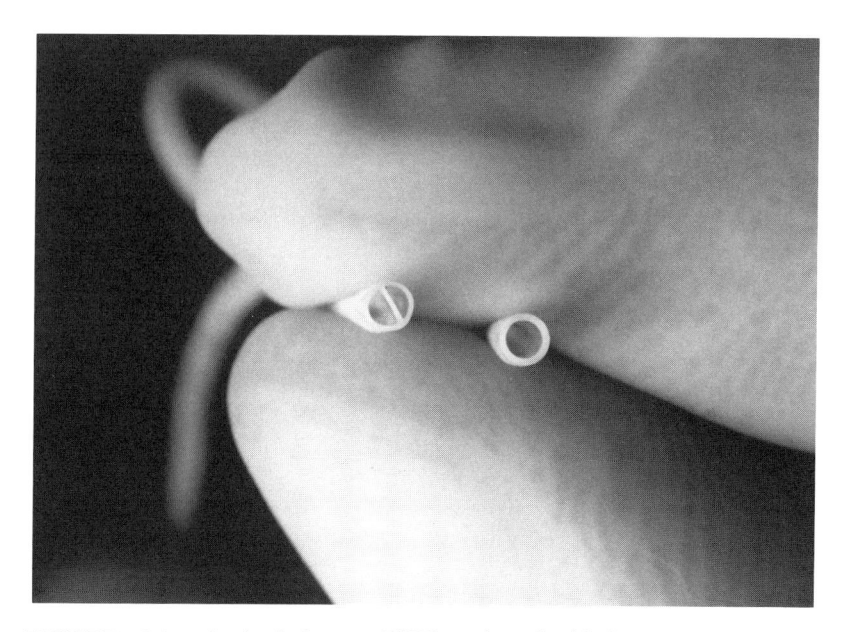

FIGURE 8-3. A single-lumen PICC and a double-lumen PICC with a "Double-D" configuration with one lumen slightly larger than the other. Note the relatively thin wall of these catheters in light of the lumen size compared to centrally placed silastic catheters.

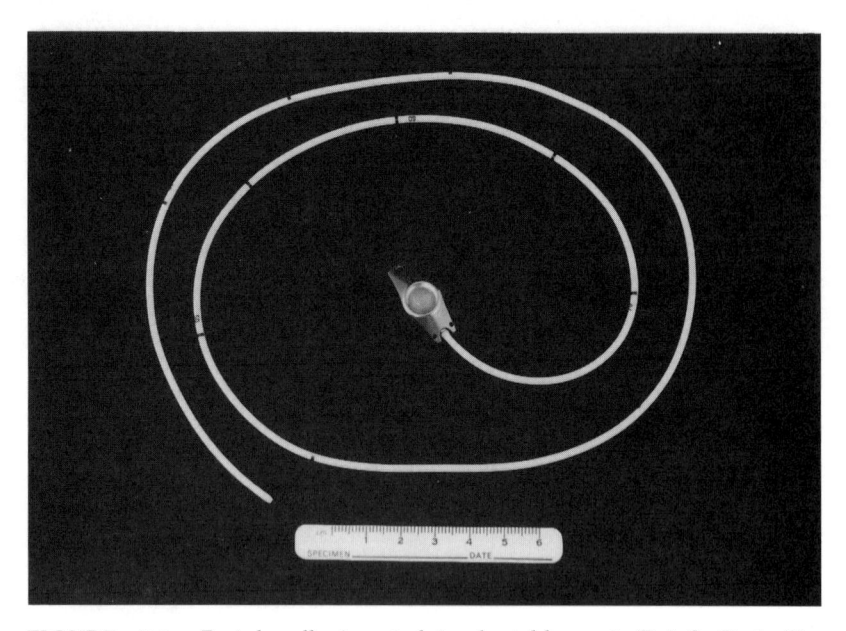

FIGURE 8-4. Peripherally inserted implantable port (P.A.S. Port, Pharmacia Deltec, St. Paul, MN). The catheter comes detached from the port housing and is connected after the tip has been positioned within the superior vena cava. The port housing should be slightly offset from the venous cutdown site so that it does not lie directly underneath the incision. This lessens the possibility of extrusion and makes subsequent access less painful.

erally implanted port, represents the combination of two previously developed technologies-the implantable port and the PICC line. The P.A.S. Port (Pharmacia Deltec, Inc., St. Paul, MN) is an example of this new device designed for peripheral placement in the arm (Figure 8-4). The port reservoir is much smaller than a low profile or standard port (Figure 8-5) and the design is intended to minimize the possibility of extrusion through the relatively scant amount of subcutaneous tissue on the forearm. The port is 10 mm high and has a septum diameter of 6.6 mm (Figure 8-6).[2] As with centrally inserted implantable ports, it is cosmetically appealing, does not interfere with lifestyle, is completely contained under the skin, and requires no bandage when not in use. An early trial with these devices found the performance to be similar to that of the standard venous chest ports. However, the manufacturer recommends that a 19-gauge access needle not be used, as this may damage the small septum.[3] A drawback to this device is the decreased area of skin rotation sites available for continuous access owing to the smaller septum size. Because this is a single-lumen device, patients requiring multiple concurrent fluids should not receive a peripheral port. Some advantages of this device include less exposure for the patient (chest exposure vs arm exposure), less magnetic resonance imaging (MRI) distortion, and lack of field obstruction during chest wall irradiation.

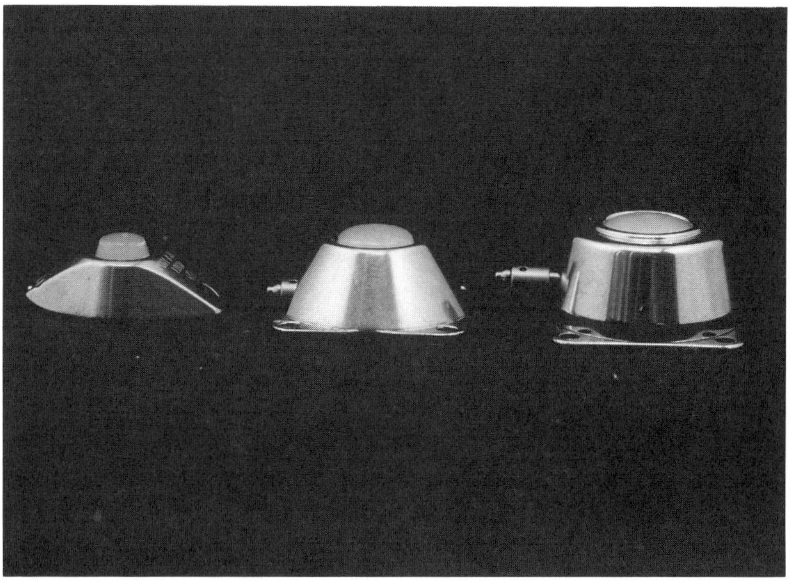

FIGURE 8-5. The three types of implantable port housings include the peripheral port *(left)*, low-profile or pediatric *(middle)* port, and the standard port *(right)*.

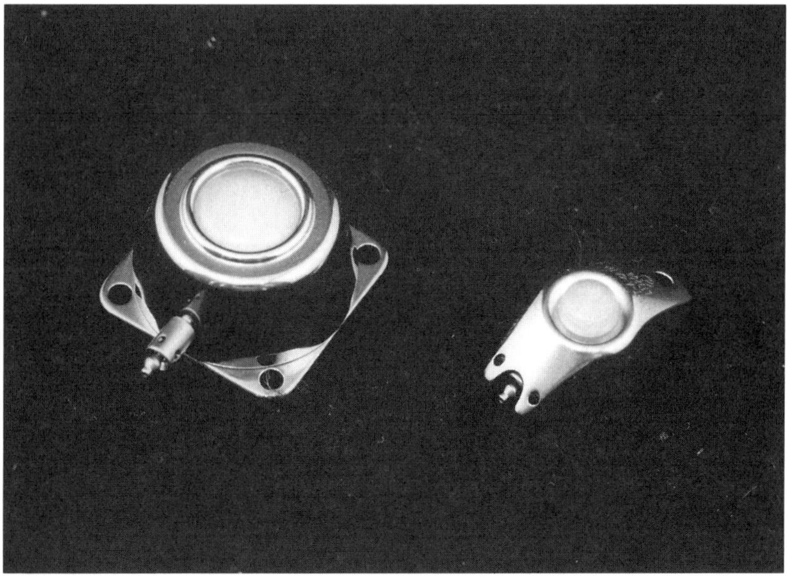

FIGURE 8-6. The profile of the peripheral port *(right)* demonstrates its design to minimize the possibility of extrusion.

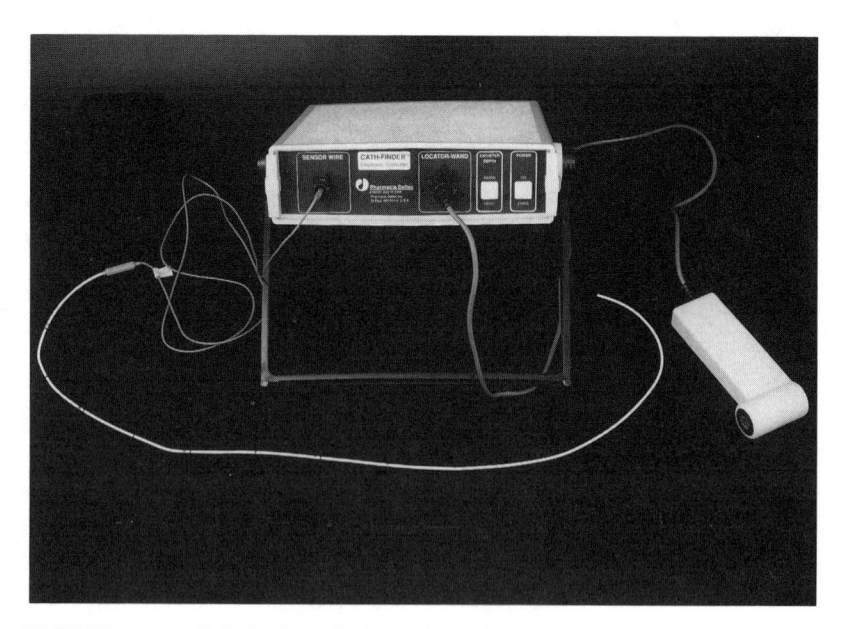

FIGURE 8-7. P.A.S. Port Cath-Finder (Pharmacia Deltec, St. Paul, MN). The Cathfinder is connected to the sensing wire that is positioned within the catheter.

Catheter Tracking Devices

The P.A.S. Port employs an electromagnetic method of tracking the catheter location called the Cath-Finder (Pharmacia Deltec, Inc., St. Paul, MN) which eliminates the need for intraoperative fluoroscopy (Figure 8-7). A guidewire that is positioned within the catheter lumen contains a sensor at the tip that emits a small amount of electromagnetic energy. A locator wand passed over the patient's precordium during placement will approximately sense the location of the catheter tip position. Although it is not a precise method of location, it can certainly discriminate a catheter positioned in the superior vena cava from one in the neck or contralateral subclavian vein. It offers the great advantages of speed and ease of use and eliminates radiation exposure and the resources required for standard fluoroscopy. However, a post-insertion chest x-ray is recommended to verify catheter tip location before the device is used.

Technique of Insertion

Because PICCs are most frequently inserted at the bedside, at home or in the clinic, attention to aseptic technique is essential. Most PICCs are available with a procedure tray that contains the equipment necessary for insertion. The patient is positioned supine with the arm designated for insertion abducted and the head turned to the ipsilateral side (Figure 8-8). The catheter length should be estimated prior to insertion by holding the catheter over its anticipated course into the cephalic or basilic vein and through the axillary and subclavian vein into the superior vena cava. In general, the catheter length will be slightly longer when inserted from the left side vs the right and a guide to assessing proper PICC length according to patient height is shown in Table 8-1.[4] After the patient's antecubital fossa has been carefully prepped and draped a percutaneous venipuncture is made into the selected vein. Because many patients have a history of repeated venipuncture or multiple previous peripheral access catheters, the identification of the basilic or cephalic vein may be difficult. In this situation a blood pressure cuff inflated to 10 to 20 mm Hg may provide the optimal conditions for venous distension. Markel and Reynen have reviewed the experience with 130 PICCs inserted at different centers.[5] In patients ranging in age from 8 to 93 years and with a variety of diagnoses, a PICC was successfully inserted on the first attempt in almost 80% and overall in 95% with two or more attempts.

There are two basic types of insertion techniques that are used and selection may be based on the operator's familiarity with either one (Figure 8-9). The first technique employs a peel away sheath comparable to that used in centrally placed long-term venous access.

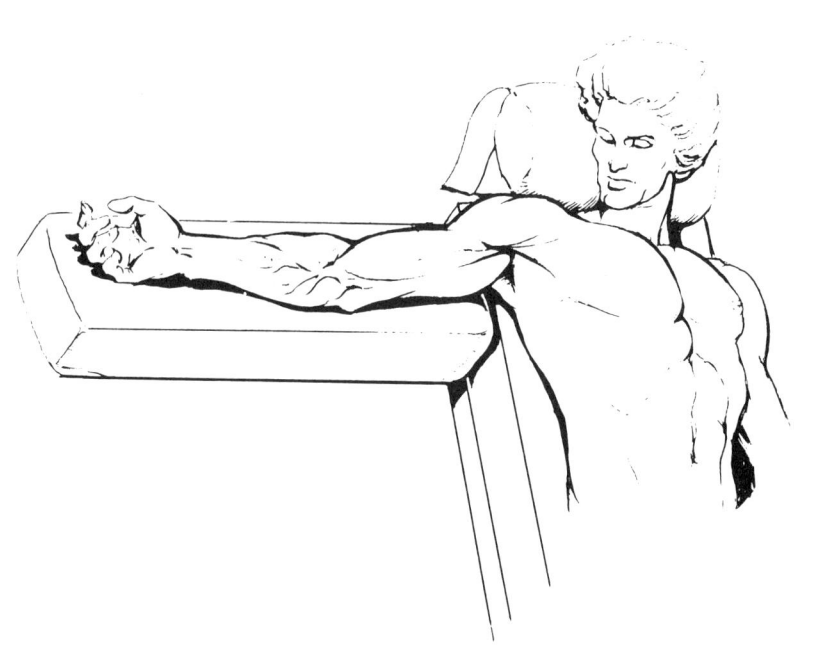

FIGURE 8-8. Typical position of a patient for placement of a PICC. The arm is abducted and the head turned to the ipsilateral side with the chin bent slightly downward.

138 Vascular Access in the Cancer Patient

TABLE 8-1
Guidelines for Estimating Appropriate Length of PICCs

Patient Height	PICC Length (cm)
5'	44
5'1"	45
5'2"	46
5'3"	47
5'4"	48
5'5"	49
5'6"–5'10"	50
5'11"	52
6'	55
6'1"	58
6'2" and over	60

Adapted from Goodwin ML. The Seldinger Method for PICC insertion. J Intraven Nurs 1989;12:238.

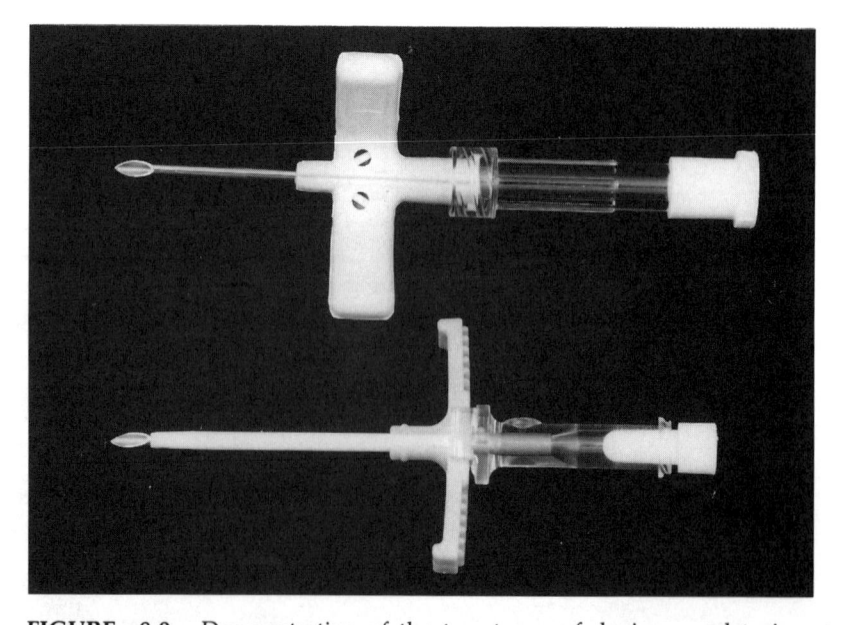

FIGURE 8-9. Demonstration of the two types of devices used to insert PICCs. The top device is a breakaway needle that is initially inserted into the vein and through which the PICC is inserted. The bottom device resembles a standard peripheral venous catheter however, the outer cannula is actually a peel away sheath similar in design to the centrally inserted peelaway sheath and through which the PICC is inserted after the needle is withdrawn.

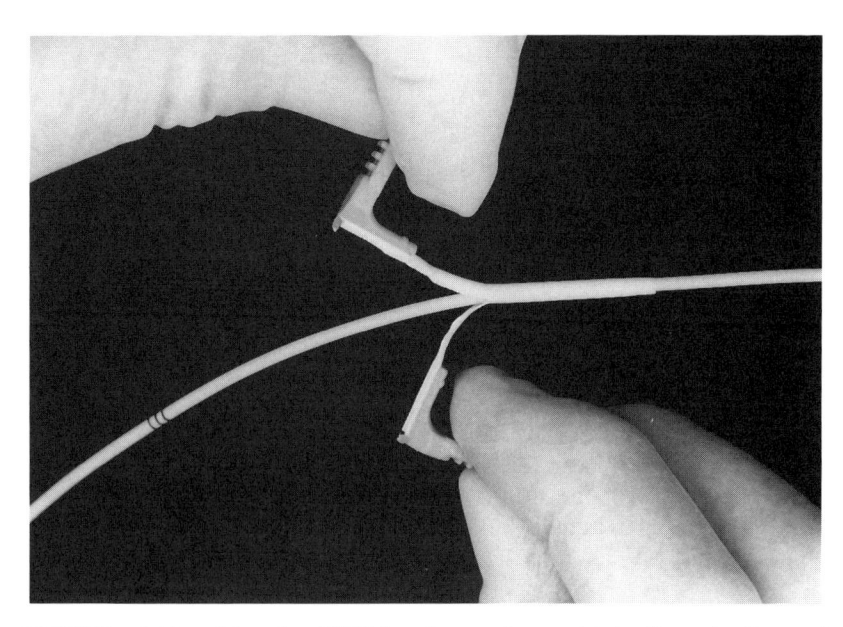

FIGURE 8-10. After the PICC has been advanced into the vein the peel away sheath is removed as shown.

A peel away sheath is advanced into the vein over a needle and the needle is then withdrawn much like a peripheral venous cannula is placed. The PICC is then inserted through the peel away sheath and advanced into the vein. The peel away sheath is then split and withdrawn out of the vein (Figure 8-10). The second technique employs a newly developed introducer needle that is initially advanced into the vein. The PICC is advanced directly through the needle which is then completely withdrawn from the vein. It is split by compressing the needle wings and separating the needle halves (Figure 8-11). After the catheter has been advanced to the appropriate location it is secured in place with sutures or steri-strips and a dry sterile dressing is applied to it. An x-ray film should be obtained to confirm final tip placement. Some have advocated a heating pad around the insertion site for 48 hours to help resolve vein irritation.[4]

When inserting a P.A.S. Port a subcutaneous pocket must be made just adjacent to the insertion site to accommodate the port housing. The port should be placed in the subcutaneous tissue and anchored in place with permanent sutures placed through the underlying muscle fascia to prevent port malposition. If excess catheter is left in the subcutaneous tissue then kinking of the catheter will be possible with movement of the arm.

Text continues on page 140

140 Vascular Access in the Cancer Patient

a

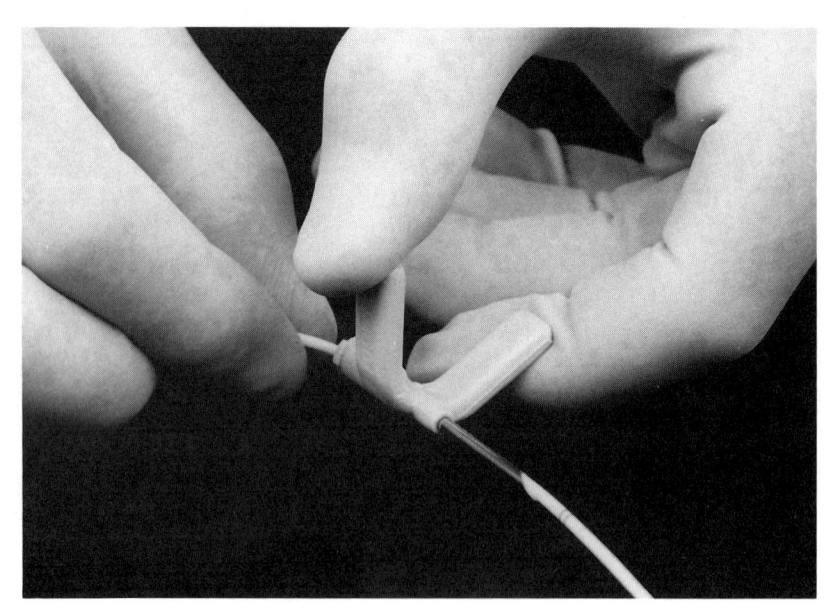

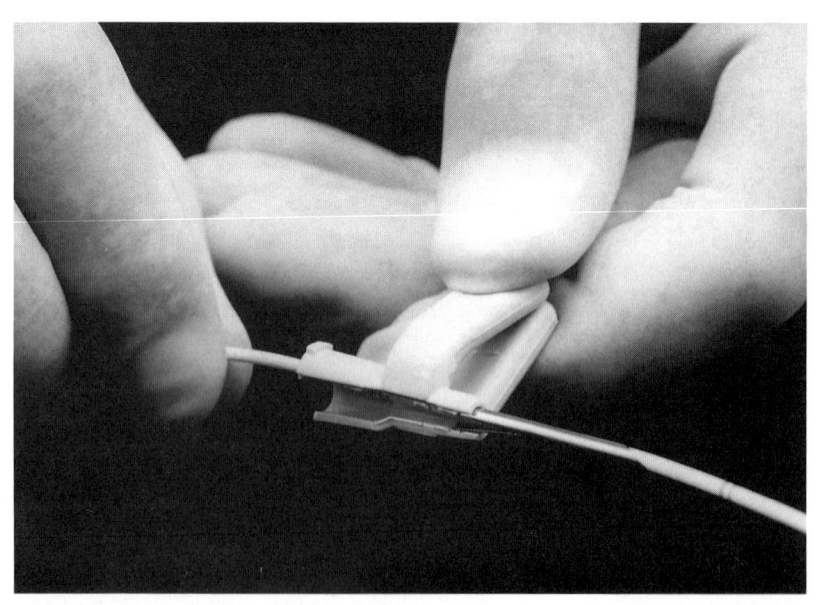

b

FIGURE 8-11. After the PICC has been inserted through the breakaway needle, the needle is withdrawn from the vein and the flanges pinched (a and b). The flanges are then snapped in the opposite direction to completely break the needle away from the catheter (c and d).

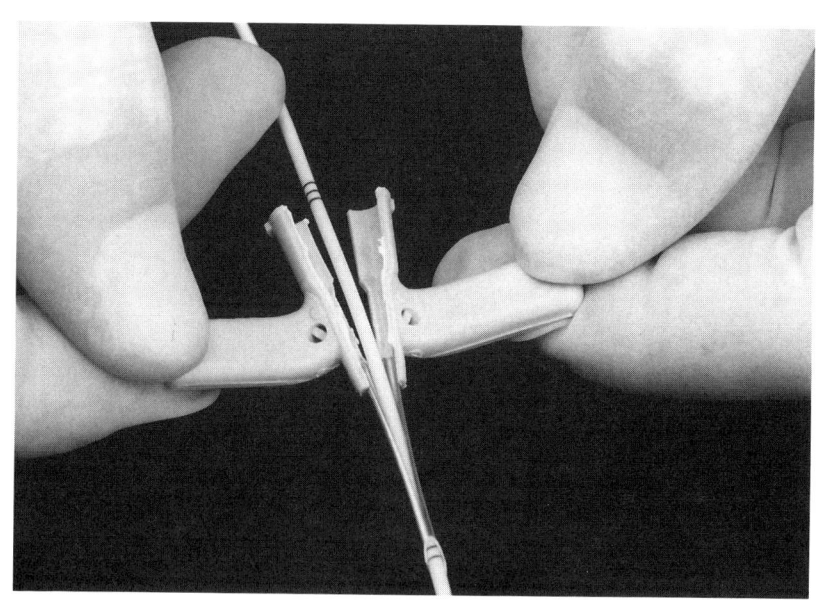

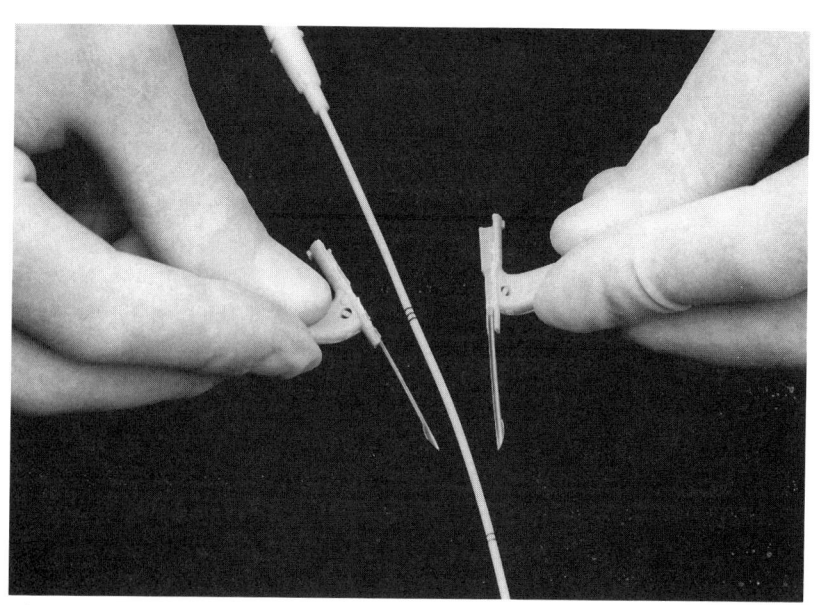

FIGURE 8-11. *Continued*

Clinical Performance of PICCs

James et al have reported experience with over 150 PICCs inserted at a single institution by a trained team of nurses.[6] Patients varied according to age and diagnosis and the average duration of catheterization was 16 days. When insertion sites were compared to determine which peripheral forearm vein might provide the best possibility of positioning the cannula into the superior vena cava, James noted the overall success rate on first insertion was 73%. Although there was no significant difference in the successful insertion rate based on site, the right basilic vein was the lowest with 68% placed within the SVC on first insertion and the left cephalic was highest (80%). The authors note that removal of the guidewire is often helpful in repositioning a catheter. Other maneuvers that were attempted included placing the patient in semi-Fowler's position or rapid push of 10 mL of saline through the catheter.

The overall complication rate of the catheters was 14.5%. The effect of a catheter within a relatively small vein and the motion of the arm appear to have a great effect on the types of complications seen with these devices. Almost four fifths of the reversible complications in this study were due to mechanical phlebitis that resolved with local treatment. Others have noted that mechanical phlebitis occurs almost exclusively in the first week after placement when endothelial injury is new.[7] Other complications reported by James et al included one clotted cannula, one ruptured cannula, one intractable phlebitis, and one vein thrombosis (Table 8-2).

Raad et al have reported the clinical results of 154 PICCs inserted into cancer patients at the M.D. Anderson Cancer Center.[8] Table 8-2 summarizes the performance profile in this study. Of note, the infection rate per 100 catheter use days (0.19) is comparable to that of Hickman-type vascular access devices (Table 8-3). When the total cost of catheter insertion and maintenance is considered on a monthly basis, PICCs appear to provide a very cost-effective alternative to tunneled venous access catheters (Table 8-4). Velardi et al have similarly noted a tenfold cost advantage using PICCs inserted in an ambulatory setting in 28 adult male patients.[9] Complications included one failed insertion attempt, two inadvertent removals, three catheter occlusions secondary to improper maintenance, and one removed early due to patient intolerance.

In the home setting PICCs may be associated with a higher incidence of complications. Graham et al have reported on the outcomes of 76 PICCs placed in patients for home-based therapy.[10] The duration of catheterization was 24 days and the PICCs were successfully used until completion of therapy in 67% of patients. However, complications were not inconsequential and included catheter clots in 16 (21%), phlebitis in 11 (14%), catheter fracture in 6 (8%), holes in 5 (7%), and accidental removal in 2 (3%). One patient experienced a line

TABLE 8-2
Selected Reviews Demonstrating the Efficacy and Complications Associated with PICCs

Author	N	Percentage Successfully Inserted and Positioned	Mean Duration	Complications, N (%)				
				Overall	Phlebitis	Occlusion	Thrombosis	Infection
James et al[6]	157	80%*	16 days	23 (14.5)	18 (11)	1	1	1
Raad et al[8]	154	N/A	87 days	71 (46)	40 (26)	—	—	25
Kyle and Myers[16]	25	92	20 days	—	2 (8)	—	—	(16)[†]
Brown[1]	26	100	13 days	8 (32)	1 (4)	—	—	0
Markel and Reynen[5]	130	95[‡]	20 days	48 (37)	5 (4)	18 (14)	—	0
Morris et al[13]	22	90	120 days	5 (23)	1 (5)	0	—	1
Graham et al[10]	76	N/A	24 days	40 (53)	11 (14)	16 (21)	0	1 (5)
Winters et al[3]	32	94	153 days	19 (59)	4 (12.5)	10 (19)	2 (6)	1 (3)

*Includes 11 patients in whom the catheter was successfully repositioned after initial insertion.
[†]Includes rate of catheter-related bacteremia, catheter colonization, and exit site purulence.
[‡]Includes 17% of patients requiring two or more insertion attempts.

TABLE 8-3
Clinical Performance of 154 PICCs Inserted at a Single Institution with Special Reference to Infection

Parameter	N (%)
PICCs	154
Mean duration, days	87
Catheter infections	25 (16)
Exit site inflammation	40 (26)
Catheter-related bacteremia	6 (3.9)
Infection rate/100 days	0.19

Modified from Raad I, Davis S, Becker M, et al. Low infection rate and long durability of nontunneled silastic catheters. Arch Intern Med 1993;153:1791–1796.

fracture with migration of a catheter segment into the pulmonary artery that ultimately required thoracotomy to retrieve.

Clinical Performance of Peripherally Implanted Ports

Several studies have recently been published reviewing the clinical performance characteristics of a peripherally inserted implantable port. Winters et al have reported the results of a prospective study evaluating the efficacy of the peripherally inserted P.A.S. Port (Pharmacia Deltec, St. Paul, MN).[3] Over a 13-month period 32 devices were inserted in adults with a variety of diagnoses and followed for complications and performance for a total of 4896 catheter use days (mean duration 153 days). Two catheters could not be placed and patients went on to receive centrally inserted ports. A summary of the 19

TABLE 8-4
Estimated Monthly Cost Savings by Using a PICC vs a Standard Long-Term Venous Access Catheter

Parameter	PICC	Long-Term Venous Access Device
Physician	—	$750
Clinic	$90	$39
Catheter	$71	$51–$161
Supplies	$21	$56–$303
Chest X-ray	$71	$71–$127
Laboratory studies	$47	$47
Flouroscopy	—	$81
Anesthesia monitoring	—	$761
OR/Recovery room	—	$217
Total	$300	$2814–$3227

Modified from Raad I, Davis S, Becker M, et al. Low infection rate and long durability of nontunneled silastic catheters. Arch Intern Med 1993;153:1791–1796.

TABLE 8-5
Complications Associated with Use of the P.A.S. Port in 32 Adult Patients

Complication	N	Percentage of Patients	Rate (per 1000 Catheter Use Days)
Malposition	1	3	0.2
Catheter occlusion	10	19	2
Pocket cellulitis	1	3	0.2
Pocket infection	1	3	0.2
Vein phlebitis	4	12.5	0.8
Vessel thrombosis	2	6	4
Total	19	44	3.88

complications occurring in 14 patients is presented in Table 8-5. Of note there were no port extrusions or extravasation due to access needle dislodgment. The authors felt that patient acceptance was very good and that the devices performed comparably to centrally accessed ports. McKee has noted an even lower rate of complications associated with P.A.S. Ports.[11] In 28 adult patients with P.A.S. Ports in for an average of 171 days, there were no catheter occlusions or vessel thromboses noted resulting in a total complication rate of 0.6/1000 catheter use days. Finney et al have reported the largest series of P.A.S. Ports in which 79 patients ranging in age from 3 to 92 years underwent bedside placement of the devices.[12] Eight (10%) patients developed superficial phlebitis that resolved within 48 hours and seven (9%) had the device removed secondary to infection. Of note, the device was successfully implanted in three patients who were fully anticoagulated without apparent adverse effect. Morris et al have reported a very low rate of significant complications in 22 peripheral ports in place for a mean of 17.6 weeks.[13] Of note, withdrawal occlusion occurred in only three patients (14%) and there was only one port pocket infection.

A second device that is designed to be placed in an interventional radiology suite has been introduced (Periport, Infusaid, Norwood, MA). Results are comparable to those observed with the P.A.S. Port. Andrews et al reported that in 35 patients with the device blood sampling was successful in almost 99% of attempts.[14]

Overall, the data show that the use of PICCs, either external devices or implanted ports, are associated with a high rate of successful insertion in selected patients that appears to increase with experience, a low incidence of complications, high patient acceptance, and relatively low cost compared to conventional centrally placed vascular access devices.[1,4,5,9,15,16] In addition, they can be placed at the bedside which eliminates the need to use operating and recovery room resources and appear to have substantial durability, as many reviews report an average dwell duration in excess of 4 months.[4,5,9]

References

1. Brown JM. Peripherally inserted central catheters: use in home care. J Intraven Nurs 1989;12:144–150.
2. P.A.S. Port-Implantable Access System, pp. 1–8. St. Paul, MN: Pharmacia Deltec Inc, 1992.
3. Winters V, Peters B, Coila S, et al. A trial with a new peripheral implanted vascular access device. Oncol Nurs Forum 1990;17:891–896.
4. Goodwin ML. The Seldinger method for PICC insertion. J Intraven Nurs 1989;12:238–243.
5. Markel S, Reynen K. Impact on patient care: 2652 PIC catheter days in the alternative setting. J Intraven Nurs 1990;13:347–351.
6. James L, Bledsoe L, Hadaway LC. A retrospective loop at tip location and complications of peripherally inserted central catheter lines. J Intraven Nurs 1993;16:104–109.
7. Hadaway LC. An overview of vascular access devices inserted via the antecubital area. J Intraven Nurs 1990;13:297–306.
8. Raad I, Davis S, Becker M, et al. Low infection rate and long durability of nontunneled Silastic catheters. Arch Intern Med 1993;153:1791–1796.
9. Velardi M, France K, Roemeling R, et al. Usefulness of Per-Q-Cath as an intermediate access device to facilitate ambulatory chemotherapy. Proc Am Soc Clin Oncol 1990;9:335.
10. Graham DR, Keldermans MM, Klemm LW, Semenza NJ, Shafer ML. Infectious complications among patients receiving home intravenous therapy with peripheral, central, or peripherally placed central venous catheters. Am J Med 1991;91:3B95S–3B100S.
11. McKee J. Future dimensions in vascular access. Peripheral implantable ports. J Intraven Nurs 1991;14:387–393.
12. Finney R, Albrink MH, Hart MB, Rosemurgy AS. A cost-effective peripheral venous port system placed at the bedside. J Surg Res 1992;53:17–19.
13. Morris P, Buller R, Kendall S, Anderson B. A peripherally implanted permanent central venous access device. Obstet Gynecol 1991;78:1138–1142.
14. Andrews JC, Walker-Andrews SC, Ensminger WD. Long-term central venous access with a peripherally placed subcutaneous infusion port: initial results. Radiology 1990;176:45–47.
15. Masoorli S, Angeles T. PICC lines: the latest home care challenge. RN 1990;15:44–51.
16. Kyle K, Myers J. Peripherally inserted central catheters: development of a hospital-based program. J Intraven Nurs 1990;13:287–290.

9
Routine Maintenance and Care of Long-Term Vascular Access Devices

Alice B. Lucas

Special Considerations with Implantable Ports
Postoperative Management of Vascular Access Devices
Device Care Issues
Routine Maintenance of External Catheters
Catheter Exit Site Care and Dressing Changes
Port Accession
Prevention of Complications
Infection Prophylaxis
Management of Complications
Education Issues
References

A wide variety of venous access devices are available, with new devices and modifications of old devices being introduced into the market almost continually. The health care professional is challenged to maintain current knowledge of the differences between the devices, the device of choice for individual patients, insertion procedures, and device maintenance protocols. Although all long-term vascular access devices serve basically the same purpose, the patient's underlying condition and type of treatment will determine which one is appropriate for insertion. It is important to recognize the advantages, limitations, and potential morbidity associated with each type of device. Matching a high-maintenance device to a noncompliant patient will ensure failure. Planning in anticipation of long-term needs will enable early placement and may decrease complications secondary to therapy administration via impaired peripheral veins.[1] There are basically two types of long-term devices, the external right atrial silastic catheter and the totally implanted venous access port.

Tunneled, cuffed silastic catheters, first described by Broviac[2] and subsequently modified by Hickman[3] were developed in the early 1970s for long-term venous access. Another variety of the dual-lumen silastic catheter that is coming into widespread use is designed to facilitate plasmapheresis, stem cell pheresis, and hemodialysis. It is similar to the Hickman-type catheter except that the tips of this catheter are staggered, the length of the external segment is shorter, and the diameters of the lumens are larger to allow for the pheresis or dialysis.

First available in 1982, totally implanted subcutaneous access ports offer a viable alternative to the right atrial silastic catheter in some patient populations and are associated with a relatively low morbidity rate when evaluated for their duration in place in the body.[4-8] Ports require essentially no patient maintenance or change in daily life activities. When the port is not accessed, it is fairly inconspicuous, visible only as a bump under the skin. This minimizes disruption in body image and allows complete freedom of activity. Ports are easily accessed by insertion of a noncoring Huber point needle through the silicone septum into the reservoir (Figure 9-1).

Special Considerations with Implantable Ports

Because a subcutaneous connection between the reservoir and the external tubing must be made each time access is desired, ports introduce a risk of drug extravasation not seen with Hickman-type catheters. The potential degree of tissue damage depends on the amount of drug absorbed, the duration of exposure, and the site of the extravasation. Because the site of the majority of implantable ports is the anterior chest, the underlying tissues and structures may be damaged. When a vesicant extravasates, the most common reaction observed is intense skin inflammation ranging from erythema of the

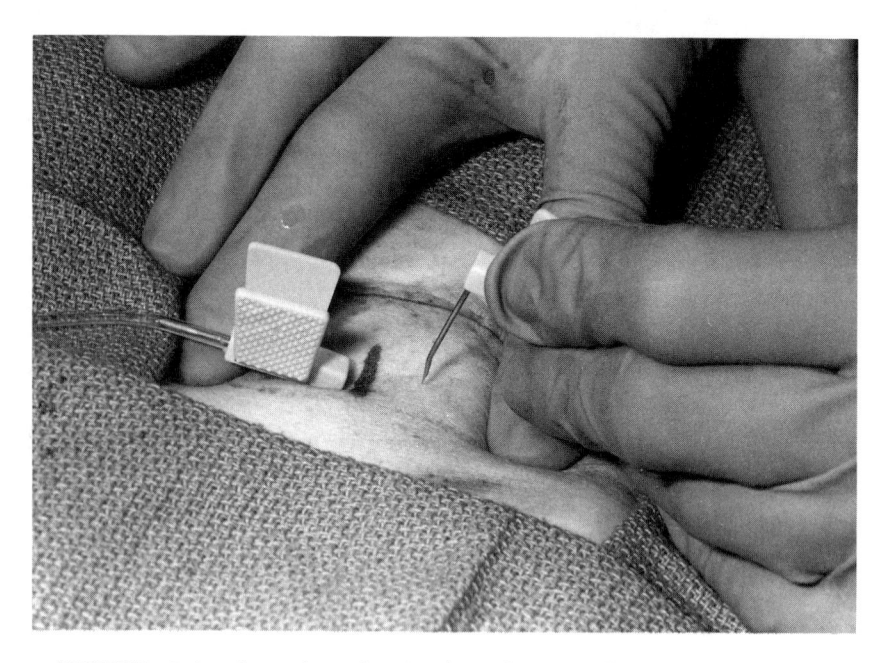

FIGURE 9-1. Accession of an implanted port with a Huber point needle.

epidermis to ulceration of subcutaneous tissues with resultant necrosis. Ulcers appear approximately 1 to 2 weeks after extravasation and may require surgical procedures to repair.[9] When this type of therapy is anticipated, an external catheter may be more appropriate. For any type of continuous outpatient infusion through a port, the patient must be instructed to monitor the site frequently for needle dislodgement, extravasation, and signs of site irritation or infection. In general, implantable ports should be used whenever clinically feasible, as they appear to be associated with less morbidity than catheters.[10–15]

Postoperative Management of Vascular Access Devices

Most long-term venous access devices are inserted under fluoroscopic guidance. A routine follow-up chest x-ray film verifies that the position of the catheter has not changed and also rules out any other insertion complications such as pneumothorax.

Expected physical findings in the immediate postoperative period include tenderness and/or pain at the incision sites and along the catheter tunnel, neck soreness secondary to positioning for placement, swelling, and accumulation of serous fluid subcutaneously surrounding the implanted port, and development of minor hematomas in thrombocytopenic patients. Patients should be offered pain medication to ease symptoms. Reports of continued pain after 2 to 3 days should be investigated. Excessive bleeding or swelling, inflammation of the catheter tunnel tract, or change in patients' vital signs should be fully evaluated.

The assessment of a peripherally inserted central catheter line site is similar to the assessment of any other type of venipuncture site. The site should be assessed at regular intervals for redness, edema, pain, drainage, or the development of a venous cord. Sutures or steristrips are used to secure the catheter to the skin insertion site. This catheter is fragile and requires a secure dressing. The dressings should be changed with the same frequency and vigilance as applied to any other central venous catheter. Exercise of the arm in which the catheter is inserted should be avoided because the contraction of the biceps muscle may create enough pressure to cause the catheter to become displaced. Small syringes should not be used to irrigate these catheters because the increased pressure may lead to catheter leaks or rupture. The pressure per square inch exerted by any electronic infusion devices used should be checked to ensure that it does not exceed the catheter recommendations. When irrigating the catheter, the first 1 to 2 mL should be flushed through gently to establish patency, with the remainder flushed vigorously to prevent buildup of fibrin or red cells in the catheter lumen.

Device Care Issues

Venous access devices require routine care to maintain their function. Review of the literature reveals few research-based protocols to support a definitive policy or procedure for device care. Controversies include volume and dose of heparin to maintain patency; frequency of heparinization to maintain patency; type of exit site dressing; frequency of dressing changes; frequency of cap changes; use of sterile or unsterile gloves for catheter care; use of masks; and choice of cleansing solutions for site care and catheter care.

Regardless of the protocol used, it is imperative that a standard procedure be adopted by the institution and followed by everyone who cares for the patient. This will provide consistency of care, prevent poor technique, and reinforce teaching for the patient. The guiding principle for all care is based on the fact that these are central catheters and because of the potential for serious, even life-threatening complications, it is important that we teach and practice a profound respect for all aspects of these devices.[16]

Routine Maintenance of External Catheters

External catheters require meticulous, frequent, and time-consuming home maintenance procedures. Consideration must be given to the patient/family's physical and intellectual ability to meet these care requirements before the catheter is inserted. Factors such as altered body image related to the catheter and impact of the catheter on the patients' lifestyle must also be given consideration in terms of how they will affect the patient's willingness to perform necessary care.

Routine maintenance of external catheters involves irrigation of each catheter lumen, injection cap change, exit site skin care, and dressing change. As stated, research is limited but general guidelines exist based on clinical experience and judgment considering the patient population, risk factors, and known complications of invasive devices and cancer treatment. The Hickman/Broviac-type catheters have traditionally required frequent flushing, generally ranging from every 12 hours while the patient is in the hospital to daily or every other day while at home.[1,10,17,18] There have been no controlled studies published indicating that this is necessary to maintain patency of the catheter. It is hypothesized that the frequency of catheter manipulation is directly correlated to the risk of catheter-related infection. At Memorial Sloan-Kettering Cancer Center a prospective evaluation was undertaken to compare the incidence of catheter-related bacteremia when patients irrigated their catheters at home when not in continual use daily as opposed to decreasing the frequency of irrigation to twice weekly.[19] The irrigation solution used (5 mL heparinized saline, 10 U/mL) was unchanged. The results of the evaluation showed a 33% decrease in the incidence of catheter-related bacteremia after the switch to twice weekly irrigation, without any increase in the incidence of vessel thrombosis or intraluminal clotting (Table 9-1). Further studies will be conducted to determine the efficacy of deceasing the frequency to once per week or perhaps changing the irrigation solution to include a routine flush with a thrombolytic agent (eg, urokinase) to decrease the risk of fibrin sheath or intraluminal clot formation.[20]

Another controversy in the management of vascular access devices is the administration of an antibiotic flush, specifically vancomycin, on a routine basis to prevent luminal colonization with vancomycin-sensitive bacteria. One study[21] confirmed that a dilute solution of vancomycin and heparin retains antibacterial and anticoagulant activities. The authors concluded that this solution may be of use in preventing catheter-related infections in patients requiring tunneled central venous catheters if it were used in place of the stan-

TABLE 9-1
Morbidity Related to Frequency of Heparinized Saline Flush

Daily Flush		Twice Weekly
985	No. of catheters	592
163,571	No. of catheter use days	87,226
396	No. of catheter-related bacteremias (CRB)*	141
18	No. of thromboses	9
103	No. of intraluminal clots	48
.0024	No. of CRB† per catheter use day*	.0016

*$P<.001$.
†CRB = catheter related bacteremia

dard heparin flush solution. Because the drug would be undetectable when flushed into the bloodstream, they felt that the selection of resistant organisms was unlikely to occur. A prospective study of 45 pediatric patients with oncologic or hematologic disorders requiring tunneled central venous catheters randomized to receive either a standard heparin flush or a vancomycin/heparin flush demonstrated that bacteremias attributed to luminal colonization with vancomycin-sensitive organisms can be prevented by using the vancomycin/heparin solution for daily flushing.[22] It will be important to replicate this study and confirm the results in a large group of patients.

The use of injection caps should be limited to when either the catheter is being used for intermittent infusions or when it is not in use at all. All continuous infusions of intravenous therapy should be directly connected to the hub of the catheter. The use of Luer lock intravenous tubing ensures a tight connection. When the injection cap is in use, it should be changed on a routine basis, generally once or twice weekly, or more often if the latex is being punctured frequently. The smallest gauge needle possible (eg, 25-gauge) should be used routinely to inject through the cap. After changing the cap, the connection should be secured with paper tape to decrease the risk of inadvertent catheter cap removal.

The Groshong right atrial silastic catheter is similar to the Hickman/Broviac-type except it has a two-way slit valve adjacent to a rounded, closed tip. Each lumen in the dual-lumen catheter has its own slit valve. The slit valve opens outward during infusion, inward during blood sample withdrawal, and closes automatically when not in use. Clamping of the catheter is unnecessary because the valve closes automatically and minimizes the risk of inadvertent infusion of air or loss of blood. When an infusion has finished, the valve closes and minimizes the risk of blood backup into the catheter. This feature eliminates the need for heparin flushes to maintain catheter patency. The catheter is irrigated with 5 mL of normal saline after each intermittent infusion and with 10 mL of normal saline after blood specimen collection or infusion of blood products. When not in use the catheter is irrigated once every 7 days with 5 mL of normal saline. Other routine maintenance is the same as for any right atrial catheter.

Catheter Exit Site Care and Dressing Changes

There is no consensus of opinion on method or type of dressing material (gauze vs transparent vs no dressing at all) in terms of patient compliance, maintenance of skin integrity, or prevention of infection. A recently published meta-analysis of the infection risks of transparent dressings when used on intravenous catheter sites created quite a controversy.[23] The authors concluded that a significantly increased risk of catheter-tip infection was demonstrated with the use of transparent compared with gauze dressings when used on intravenous catheters. They also stated that an increased risk of bacteremia and catheter sepsis associated with the use of transparent dressings on central venous catheters was suggested.

The interpretation of the results of this large meta-analysis warrants some discussion. Although this meta-analysis was published in 1992, the studies analyzed were published between 1982 and 1989 (with the majority published in 1984 and 1985) which indicates that they were actually conducted before that time period. As a result of improved quality in terms of moisture vapor permeability, the transparent dressings in use today are not comparable to the products used in these studies. The article reviews only randomized comparative studies of conventional transparent films vs tape and gauze. Thirteen studies were removed from consideration because they did not meet all of the selection criteria. The meta-analysis also did not review any of the positive studies performed using transparent films alone.

There were many factors that varied among the studies for central venous catheters including:

Brand of catheter
Location of catheter
Patient population
Clinical use of catheter
Frequency of dressing change
Skin care regimen used
Use and type of topical antibacterial ointment

With these factors not controlled, it is difficult to ascertain the actual effect of only the dressings on the risk of infection. Any one or all of these factors could significantly contribute to that risk. Utilization of the findings of the research studies to practice is challenged because of the variability of the nursing procedures, the differing lengths of time that catheters are in place, the different types of catheters used in the study, and the different brands of dressings used.

Of note the results of the meta-analysis were statistically significant in only one category, that of catheter-tip infection. This indicates that the catheter tip culture was positive but blood cultures were negative. The article provided no information about how the devices were removed, how the skin was prepped before removal, who removed the devices, and how the devices were cultured, all of which could affect the rate of contamination on catheter removal and subsequently the number of positive catheter tips. The results of the analysis in other categories of infection for example, bacteremia and catheter-related sepsis, were not statistically significant. The above referenced analysis must be interpreted carefully before any changes in clinical practice are contemplated.

In practice, transparent dressings are recommended and have been used for years on implanted ports to enable visualization of the needle insertion site without apparent or reported problems with skin

TABLE 9-2
Catheter Exit Site Dressings

Type	Advantages	Disadvantages
Transparent	Permeable membrane allows oxygen, moisture, vapor out; impermeable to bacteria. Allows visualization of site. Can remain in place four to seven days. Greater patient comfort.	Expensive. Cleansing of the site only with dressing change. Studies indicating greater colonization of bacteria. Poor adhesion with diaphoresis.
Gauze	Absorbs moisture. Less expensive.	Cleansing of the site only with dressing change. No visualization of site. Greater frequency of change – daily to every three days.
No Dressing	Daily cleansing of the site. Allows visualization of the site. No irritation related to adhesive. No expense.	Greater risk of catheter dislodgment. No barrier against contamination.

irritation or increased incidence of colonization of bacteria or infection. The relative advantages and disadvantages of different types of exit site dressings are shown in Table 9-2.

Skin care procedures range from simple cleaning with soap and water (for tunneled catheters after engraftment of the Dacron cuff)[24] to defatting the skin with alcohol before a povidone-iodine solution scrub, which is followed by application of either povidone-iodine ointment or an antimicrobial ointment. One study suggested that vigorous cleansing of the catheter exit site may destroy the skin's natural defensibility, making it vulnerable to irritation and infection.[25] Another study[26] demonstrated a trend toward more *Candida* species colonization with the use of a polymicrobial ointment. Regardless of the frequency of care, daily hygiene must be strongly encouraged to decrease colonization of skin bacteria. One prospective study noted that a sterile skin preparation technique was no more effective at removing skin flora from the access site than a clean preparative technique. The same study revealed that patients with poor hygiene were shown to have a significantly increased incidence of skin colonization of the access site with *Staphylococcus aureus* after skin preparation.[27] Because the goal is to minimize irritation to the skin surrounding the catheter exit site and maintain skin integrity, individualized care protocols based on patient assessment are appropriate. At 1 month postinsertion of tunneled catheters, if the skin is intact with good tissue granulation and without signs/symptoms of local site infection, the site is still cleansed daily, but the dressing becomes optional.[18] If the patient does not wear a dressing, the catheter must be secured to the chest in some manner (band-aid, paper tape, etc.) to prevent accidental catheter dislodgement.

Port Accession

Before accessing any subcutaneous port, it is essential to verify the type of device and the location of the attached catheter tip. Visible only as raised bumps beneath the skin, ports look the same and feel the same on palpation and are generally accessed in the same manner. Although the location of the port pocket in a particular area of the body may be helpful in identifying the purpose of the port, the truly distinguishing feature is the location of the attached catheter tip-venous, arterial, epidural, or intraperitoneal. Methods of verifying catheter tip location include review of the operative note in the patient's permanent record, radiographic report (chest x-ray film, dye study), and/or physician confirmation of placement.

A patient should return from the operating room with the port accessed and ready for use because postoperative pain and swelling may prevent access attempts for several days. The port area may be prepared with a local anesthetic to decrease sensation as the needle is inserted. The size and type of needle for access depend on the indication for use of the port. Regardless, only a Huber point noncoring needle may be used, as any other needle will damage the silicone septum and may cause it to lose its integrity prematurely. The needle should not be of a size or configuration to interfere with the visualization of the insertion site. Needles inserted for continuous infusion should be nonsiliconized with an attached administration set. For bolus infusion or single access for blood withdrawal, a siliconized needle may be used provided it is removed immediately after the procedure is completed to decrease the risk of the needle slipping out of the septum. Nonsiliconized needles may be left in place in the port septum and used for continuous infusions or heparin locked for periods of 1 to 2 weeks, depending on the patient's clinical condition. If erythema or inflammation occurs at the site, the needle should be changed. The most commonly used needle is a 20-gauge 3/4-inch right-angled needle, with a 19-gauge preferred for transfusions and a 22-gauge adequate for access in pediatric patients. Patients in whom the port is deeply implanted may require a longer needle to attain access. A newly developed alternative to the Huber needle for accessing implanted ports, the Surecath, uses an introducer spike to pass a flexible Teflon catheter through the septum into the port reservoir. When the introducer unit is removed, the 19-gauge catheter is left in place.[28]

A dressing is necessary only when the port is accessed. A transparent dressing is commonly used to allow visualization of the needle insertion site. The dressing is changed and skin care performed when the Huber needle is changed or more frequently if the dressing becomes wet or nonocclusive or there are signs of local skin irritation or infection. Skin care may consist of alcohol and/or povidone-iodine scrub, with or without application of povidone-iodine ointment or antimicrobial ointment. Individual assessment may indicate the appropriate protocol for each patient. Showering is allowed while the port is accessed if a waterproof cover is placed over the dressing.

Irrigation of the implanted port is usually performed by health care personnel either after use or routinely on a monthly basis. The port is irrigated with heparinized saline (100 U/mL) in a large enough volume to ensure clearance of both the port reservoir and the catheter lumen, usually 3 to 5 mL, unless blood specimens have been obtained through the device. In that case, the port should be irrigated with 10 to 20 mL of normal saline before heparinization to remove any residual blood cells[29,30] The policy at Memorial Sloan-Kettering Cancer Center is to irrigate the port with 5 mL of normal saline before each heparinization to clear the device of any remaining infusate. Regardless, the irrigation should be performed vigorously to maintain patency of the device. Patients who receive continuous intravenous infusions administered through a venous port in the home setting may be taught how to heparinize the port themselves when the infusion has finished.

Prevention of Complications

Relative to the number of days any of these devices are maintained in the patient's body, device morbidity is relatively small.[16] Common sense is often the key to preventing complications associated with venous access devices. Securing the catheter or intravenous tubing to the patient may prevent accidental catheter or port needle dislodgement. Scissors should never be used during any device care procedure. If resistance is met during catheter irrigation, ensure that the catheter clamp has been removed to avoid catheter rupture. Force should never be used to irrigate a port or catheter to avoid not only rupture but catheter embolization as well. Intraluminal occlusion may occur secondary to a blood clot or drug precipitate. Most blood-clotted catheters can be cleared whereas those occluded by drug precipitate usually cannot. Intraluminal clots may be prevented by adequate catheter irrigation, acknowledging completion of all infusions, and by not administering incompatible solutions simultaneously. All health care professionals need a solid knowledge base about drug and fluid compatibilities to avoid the formation of precipitates in the line which will prevent unnecessary removal of a device.

All intravenous connections should be taped or otherwise secured. When an implanted port is accessed, the patient should be instructed to limit arm movement on the side of the port, and all supplies should be placed within easy reach of the patient. When the hospitalized patient has a continuous infusion, needle placement and the port site should be assessed at least every 2 hours to detect early signs of extravasation.

Infection Prophylaxis

The prevention of catheter-related infections centers on device care which in most instances will be performed by the patient. Adequate patient education must be ensured, with an emphasis on never performing any device care in the bathroom to avoid contamination with enteric bacteria. Recent experience with antimicrobial silver-impregnated cuffs placed on nontunneled percutaneously inserted central venous catheters suggests that such a cuff may render the catheter less prone to infection.[26,31] At Memorial Sloan-Kettering Cancer Center, 200 cancer patients were prospectively randomized to receive either a standard, dual-lumen Hickman-type cuffed silastic external catheter or the same catheter with a second, more proximal subcutaneous silver-impregnated cuff. Prospective evaluation revealed no difference in the incidence of catheter-related bacteremia/fungemia or tunnel tract infection as a result of the silver cuff.[32] A complete discussion of infection prophylaxis is presented in Chapter 7.

Management of Complications

Many of the complications that do occur with venous access devices can be managed without detriment to the patient or the device. Interventions to reverse complications should be attempted in most cases before removing the device.

One commonly occurring complication is extravasation of *nonvesicant* intravenous fluid into the subcutaneous tissue surrounding the venous device. In the external catheter, this signifies a leak in the device underneath the skin and the only option is catheter removal. However, in the implanted port this occurrence is similar to a peripheral extravasation and may be treated in much the same way. The most common explanation for extravasation is the displacement of the Huber needle. If the needle is not completely out of the port septum, needle placement can be verified by applying direct pressure on the needle until contact is made with the base of the reservoir and then check for blood return. If needle verification is not possible, the existing needle should be removed, and if possible the extravasate should be gently expressed from the tissue surrounding the port. Application of warm compresses will aid in reabsorption of fluid that is not expressed. When the fluid has been expressed or reabsorbed, the port should be reaccessed.

Another cause of extravasation is damage to the integrity of the implanted port septum. In this case, gently flush the port with 10 mL of normal saline solution while observing for swelling or leakage at the site. If either is present, notify the physician. Damage of the port septum or the catheter can be confirmed by a dye study performed through the device.

Blood withdrawal occlusion is defined as the inability to draw blood through the device when it is able to be irrigated without resistance.[33] With the implanted port this may simply be caused by an incorrectly placed Huber needle with the needle bevel within the septum rather than in the port reservoir (Figure 9-2). In this case, needle placement may be verified by applying pressure on the needle until contact is made with the base, or if the needle has been placed too close to the sides of the septum rather than in the middle, the needle will have to be removed and a sterile one reinserted.

In both catheters and ports, withdrawal occlusion and catheter occlusion may be an intermittent problem. One completely preventable cause of catheter occlusion is intraluminal precipitation caused by incompatible mixtures of drugs/solutions (eg, Dilantin/D_5W). Prevention is often the only course of action, as once the drug crystals have lodged within the catheter lumen they are extremely difficult to dissolve. If drug precipitate is highly suspected, the application of warm soaks over the catheter tunnel may help reverse the crystallization.

Catheter occlusions may be attributed to precipitates of poorly soluble fluid components, such as the calcium salts in total parenteral nutrition (TPN). Although thrombolytic agents are ineffective in these circumstances, catheter patency can be restored if the solubility of the

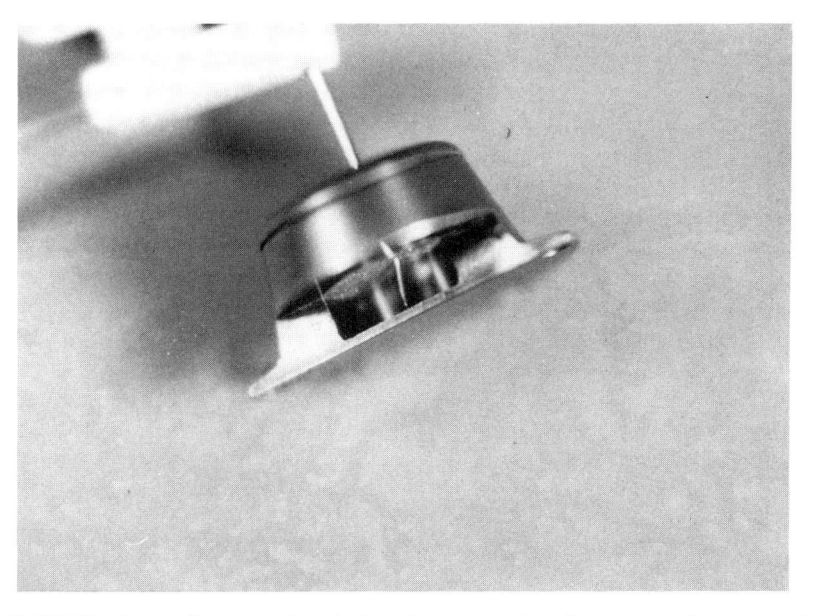

FIGURE 9-2. Cross-sectional view demonstrating the correct placement of the Huber point needle through the port septum.

fluid components is increased, for example, by lowering the pH by using 0.1N hydrochloric acid (HCl). Because of its safety, efficacy, and low cost (especially when compared with device replacement), HCl should be considered as an additional agent to clear an obstructed catheter of unknown etiology.[34] Occlusions that are caused by lipid containing solutions have been successfully cleared by the use of a 70% solution of ethanol in sterile water.[35] Information on the diagnosis and treatment of catheter occlusion is presented in Chapter 6.

Catheters are at risk for leaks or breaks in the external segment simply because they are manipulated so frequently. If a break occurs in either a single- or multi-lumen catheter, it may be repaired with the appropriate repair kit (available from the manufacturer) by specially trained nurses or physicians if the break is distant enough from the exit site to allow the repair limb to be attached to an adequate length of old catheter. These catheters have different diameters; thus repair kits are not interchangeable. Only the repair kit specifically designed for the type and diameter of the catheter should be used. Before repairing a catheter, the exit site should be inspected for signs of inflammation or infection. If the skin around the exit site is normal or minimally inflamed, the catheter may be repaired. The repair of any type of catheter is a sterile procedure. Some catheters, such as the Groshong, may be repaired using a simple replacement section that contains a stylet. After the damaged section of the catheter is removed, the replacement section is inserted into the remaining catheter, the stylet is withdrawn, and the replacement segment is snap-locked onto the catheter.

Hickman-type catheters have a much more cumbersome repair procedure. The replacement section of the catheter has a permanent metal stylet and an external sleeve that slides over the repair site. In preparation for the repair, the replacement section is primed with heparin flush solution and a syringe with a blunt needle is filled with silastic glue. After the damaged section of the catheter is removed, the metal stylet is inserted into the remaining catheter and silastic glue is applied over the repair site. The external sleeve is then slipped over the connection and more silastic glue is injected under both ends of the outer sleeve. Using a gauze pad, the outer sleeve is rolled around with the fingers to evenly distribute the glue. The repaired catheter may be used immediately; however, the connection site must be anchored with a tongue blade for 24 hours for support while the glue is drying. Chapter 1 provides additional information about catheter repair kits.

Education Issues

Education about all aspects of venous access devices including routine maintenance and management of complications is of vital concern, both to staff and the patient receiving the device. Health professionals must be well versed in all areas of device care to enable them to educate patients successfully and impress on them the importance of following the guidelines set out for them to maximize the function of their devices.

The many aspects of the home maintenance procedures may confuse and overwhelm the patient. Adequate time must be provided for teaching and questions. Ideally, teaching sessions should be conducted both before and after device insertion. The patient then knows what to expect from the procedure, what the device looks like, and how it functions and is able to become familiar with the routine maintenance requirements of the particular device to be inserted. Although there is a lack of research on the optimal way to educate patients, all of the available teaching aids should be utilized. These include videotapes, patient education booklets and cards, attendance at interactive classes, and hands-on practice using a dummy model or an actual device. As well as learning the device maintenance routine, the patient must be instructed about potential complications of the device and how to manage these complications. It is essential that the patient knows how and when to contact health care personnel in the event of a complication or a question and must also be able to distinguish between emergency and nonemergency situations.

Before the patient is discharged and considered capable of performing device care, return demonstrations must be performed and documented in the patient record. He or she must also be able to verbalize the signs/symptoms of complications that require medical attention. If it is apparent that the patient will have difficulty performing or understanding any aspect of the care, it is essential that a home health care agency be contacted to assist with the device maintenance. The patient should be provided with a medical alert identification card and/or bracelet indicating which type of venous access device is in place and its location. This should be carried at all times to identify the device in the event of an emergency. This card should also indicate resource personnel to be contacted in the event of a problem with the device.

The extent to which optimal nursing procedures could decrease the incidence of catheter-related complications has not yet been determined. Because nurses assume primary responsibility for the care of venous access devices, it is imperative for them to address the controversial issues surrounding the maintenance procedures for each type of device.

Randomized research studies need to be conducted in controlled settings for each aspect of device care. Large numbers of patients must be enrolled into these studies to ensure significance of the results. Because institutional device care policies may not take all variables into account, health care professionals must be prepared to make modifications in procedures on a case-by-case basis based on a clinical assessment of each patient.

References

1. Simon RC. Small gauge central venous catheters and right atrial catheters. Semin Oncol Nurs 1987;3:87–95.
2. Broviac JW, Schribner BH. Prolong ed parenteral nutrition in the home. Surg Gynecol Obstet 1974;139:24–28.
3. Hickman RO, Buckner CD, Clife RA, Sanders JE, Stewart P, Thomas ED. A modified right atrial catheter for access to the venous system in marrow transplant recipients. Surg Gynecol Obstet 1979;148:871–875.
4. Niederhuber JE, Ensminger W, Gyves JW, Lipeman M, Doan K, Cozzi E. Totally implanted venous and arterial access system to replace external catheters in cancer treatment. Surgery 1982;92: 706–712.
5. Strum S, McDermed J, Korn A, Joseph C. Improved methods for venous access: the Port-A-Cath, a totally implanted catheter system. J Clin Oncol 1986;4:596–603.
6. Brothers TE, Von Moll LK, Niederhuber JE, Roberts JA, Walker-Andrews S, Ensminger WD. Experience with subcutaneous infusion ports in three hundred patients. Surg Gynecol Obstet 1988; 166:295–301.
7. Grannan KJ, Taylor PH. Early and late complications of totally implantable venous access devices. J Surg Oncol 1990;44:52–54.
8. Groeger JS, Lucas A, Coit D, et al. Totally implanted venous access ports in cancer patients: a prospective evaluation of morbidity. Proc Am Soc Clin Oncol 1990;9:320.
9. Camp-Sorrell D. Implantable ports: everything you always wanted to know. J Intraven Nurs 1992;15:262–273.
10. Mirro J Jr, Rao BN, Stokes DC, et al. A prospective study of Hickman/Broviac catheters and implantable ports in pediatric oncology patients. J Clin Oncol 1989;7:214–222.
11. Mirro J Jr, Rao BN, Kumar M, et al. A comparison of placement techniques and complications of externalized catheters and implantable port use in children with cancer. J Pediatr Surg 1990; 25:120–124.
12. Groeger JS, Lucas A, Brown A. Venous access device infections in adult cancer patients: catheters vs ports. ICAAC 1988;28:158.
13. Wurzel CL, Halom K, Feldman JG, Rubin LG. Infection rates of Broviac-Hickman catheters and implantable venous devices. AJDC 1991;142:536–540.
14. Ross MN, Haase GM, Poole MA, Burrington JD, Odom LF. Comparison of totally implanted reservoirs with external catheters as venous access devices in pediatric oncologic patients. Surg Gynecol Obstet 1988;167:141–144.
15. LaQuaglia MP, Lucas A, Thaler HT, et al. A prospective analysis of vascular access device-related infections in children. J Pediatr Surg 1992;27:840–842.

16. Wachs T, Watkins S, Hickman RO. "No more pokes": a review of parenteral access devices. Nutrit Support Serv 1987;7:12–18.
17. Williard W, Coit D, Lucas A, Groeger JS. Long-term vascular access via the inferior vena cava. J Surg Oncol 1991;46:162–166.
18. Handy C. Vascular access devices: hospital to home care. J Intraven Nurs 1989;12:s10–s17.
19. Lucas AB, Groeger JS. A prospective evaluaton of Hickman catheter morbidity with twice weekly flushing compared to daily flushing. Int Consenses Support Care Oncol Belgium 1990.
20. Lawson M. Partial occlusion of inswelling central venous catheters. JIN 1991;14:157–159.
21. Henrickson KJ, Powell KR, Schwartz CL. A dilute solution of vancomycin and heparin retains antibacterial and anticoagulant activities. J Infect Dis 1988;157:600–601.
22. Schwartz C, Henrickson KJ, Roghmann K, Powell K. Prevention of bacteremia attributed to luminal colonization of tunneled central venous catheters with vancomycin-susceptible organisms. J Clin Oncol 1990;8:1591–1597.
23. Hoffman KK, Weber DJ, Samsa GP, et al. Transparent polyurethane film as an intravenous catheter dressing: a meta-analysis of the infection risks. JAMA 1992;267:2072–2076.
24. Petrosino B, Becker H, Christian B. Infection rates in central venous catheter dressings. Oncol Nurs Forum 1988;15:709–717.
25. Schwartz-Fulton J, Tischenko MM. Hickman catheter exit site skin sensitivities in an oncology patient population. NITA 1985;8:63–68.
26. Flowers RH III, Schwenzer KJ, Kopel RF, Fisch MJ, Tucker SI, Farr BM. Efficacy of an attachable subcutaneous cuff for the prevention of intravascular catheter-related infection. A randomized, controlled trial. JAMA 1989;261:878–883.
27. Kaplowitz LG, Comstock JA, Landwehr DM, et al. Prospective study of microbial colonization of the nose and skin and infection of the vascular access site in hemodialysis patients. J Clin Microbiol 1988;26:1257–1262.
28. Brown JM. Evaluation of Surecath access device. J Intraven Nurs 1989;12:298–300.
29. Goodman MS. Venous access devices: an overview. Oncol Nurs Forum 1984;11:16–23.
30. Hagle ME. Implantable devices for chemotherapy: access and delivery. Semin Oncol Nurs 1987;3:96–105.
31. Maki DG, Cobb L, Garman JK, Shapiro JM, Ringer M, Helgerson RB. An attachable silver-impregnated cuff for prevention of infection with central venous catheters: a prospective randomized multicenter trial. Am J Med 1988;85:307–314.
32. Groeger JS, Lucas AB, Coit D, et al. A prospective randomized evaluation of the effect of silver impregnated subcutaneous cuffs for preventing tunneled chronic venous access catheter infections in cancer patients. Ann Surg 1993;218:206–210.

33. Tschirhart JM, Rao MK. Mechanism and management of persistent withdrawal occlusion. Am Surg 1988;54:326–328.
34. Shulman RJ, Reed T, Pitre D, et al. Use of hydrochloric acid to clear obstructed central venous catheters. JPEN 1988;12:509–510.
35. Pennington CR, Pithie AD. Ethanol lock in the management of catheter occlusion. JPEN 1987;11:507–508.

Appendices

APPENDIX A
Considerations in Selecting the Appropriate Vascular Access Device

Vascular Access Device	Consideration*
External	• Good for prolonged infusional therapy • Less chance of extravasation versus port • Requires routine maintenance by patient
Implanted ports	• Best for intermittent/maintenance therapy • Less patient maintenance • No limitations on activity • Requires access via Huber needle
PICCs	• Good for intermediate (3–6 weeks) and possibly longer therapy • Requires adequate peripheral access • Can be inserted in home or hospice setting • Eliminates risk of central venous insertion, i.e. pneumothorax
Single-Lumen	• Less maintenance than double lumen • Less infectious complications than double lumen • Not infrequently only lumen one of a double lumen device is used
Double-lumen	• Anticipated need for second lumen • No additional risk for insertion or removal versus single-lumen • Double-lumen port housing is large
Triple-lumen	• Appropriate for intensive therapy with treatment using chemotherapy, antibiotics, TPN, transfusions, and interval blood tests

*Patient familiarity and preference should be considered in each instance.

APPENDIX B
Considerations in Selecting the Most Suitable Site for Long-Term Venous Access

Site	Consideration
Supradiaphragmatic	• Insertion sites are cleaner • Better patient acceptance • Lower risk of infectious complications • Catheter "pinch-off" possible with subclavian vein insertion
Infradiaphragmatic	• Good alternative if supradiaphragmatic sites are exhausted • Possibly higher risk of venous thrombotic complications • Multiple sites suitable such as saphenous, inferior epigastric, or direct femoral vein insertion
Supradiaphragmatic, left side	• Easier to advance due to favorable subclavian brachiocephalic vein junction • Less risk of catheter tip malposition • Possibly less risk of pneumothorax with insertion • Higher incidence of catheter-related venous thrombosis
Supradiaphragmatic, right side	• Higher risk of catheter tip malposition • Precordium is available for echocardiography • Avoids possibility of thoracic duct injury • Preferable side for internal jugular vein site
Percutaneous	• Better cosmetic result • Insertion sites reusable • Faster insertion time • Most commonly used technique
Cutdown	• Avoids possible pneumothorax • Safer for thrombocytopenic patient • More discomfort secondary to incision site • Pre-determining appropriate catheter length may be difficult • Cephalic vein insertion site can also be used for port pocket

APPENDIX C
Paradigm for the Evaluation and Treatment of Persistent Withdrawal Occlusion

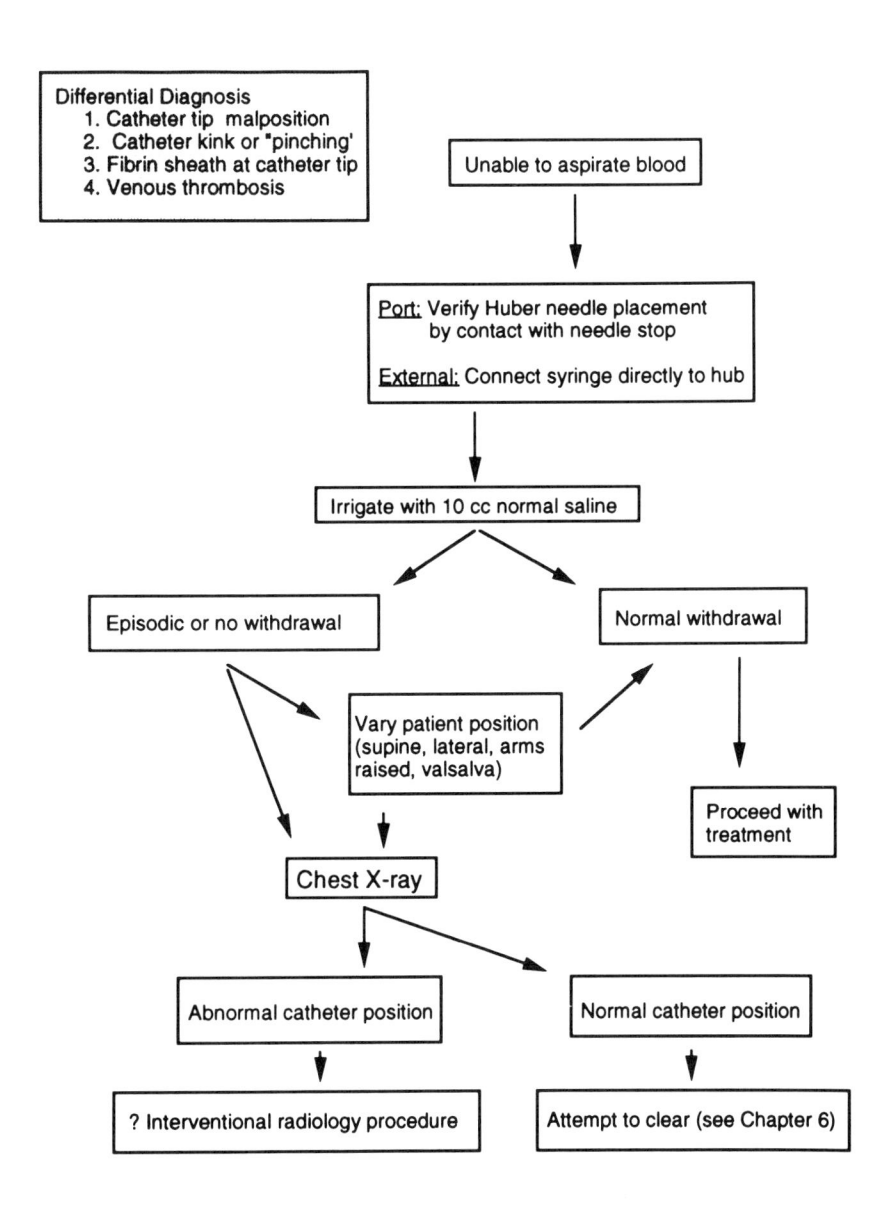

Differential Diagnosis
1. Catheter tip malposition
2. Catheter kink or "pinching"
3. Fibrin sheath at catheter tip
4. Venous thrombosis

Unable to aspirate blood
↓
Port: Verify Huber needle placement by contact with needle stop
External: Connect syringe directly to hub
↓
Irrigate with 10 cc normal saline
↓
- Episodic or no withdrawal
- Normal withdrawal → Proceed with treatment

Episodic or no withdrawal → Vary patient position (supine, lateral, arms raised, valsalva) → Normal withdrawal

Vary patient position → Chest X-ray
Episodic or no withdrawal → Chest X-ray

Chest X-ray:
- Abnormal catheter position → ? Interventional radiology procedure
- Normal catheter position → Attempt to clear (see Chapter 6)

APPENDIX D
Paradigm for the Evaluation and Treatment of Partial Catheter Occlusion

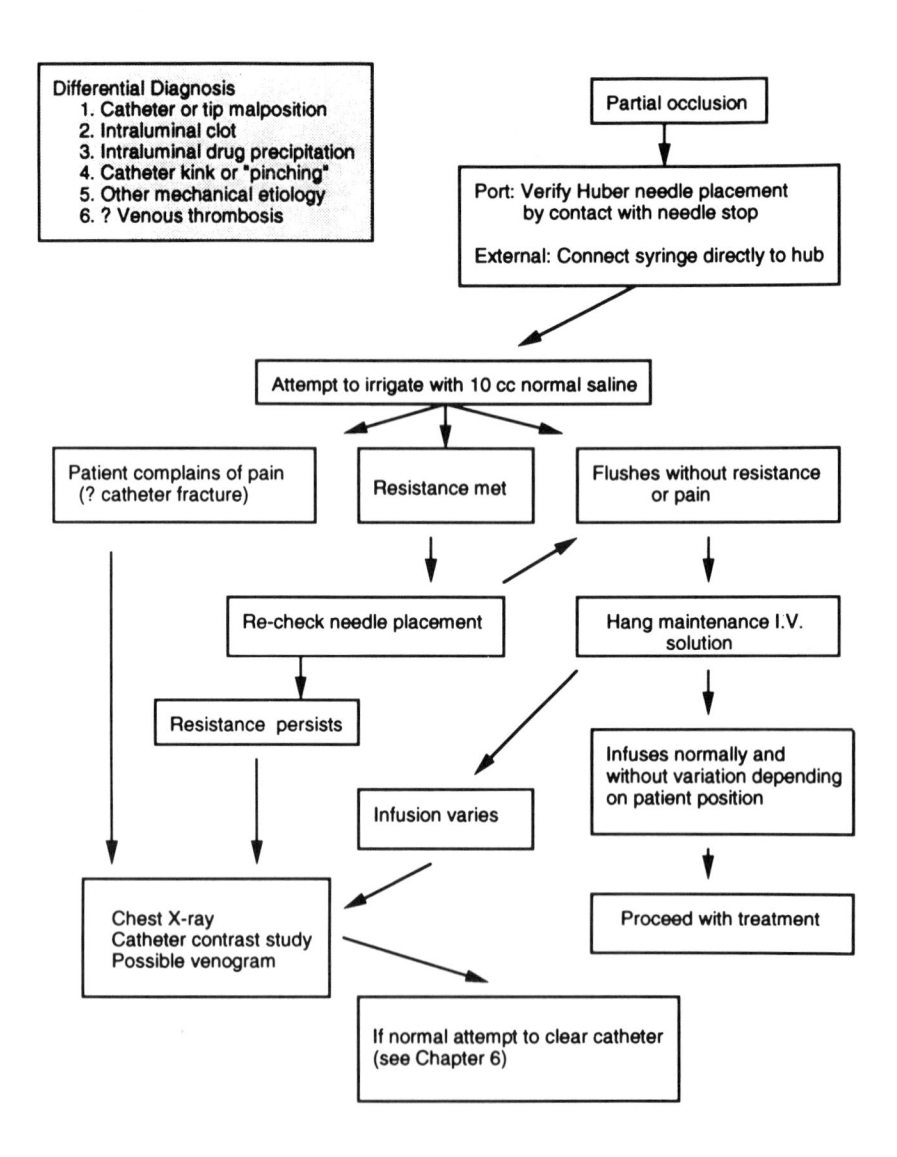

Differential Diagnosis
1. Catheter or tip malposition
2. Intraluminal clot
3. Intraluminal drug precipitation
4. Catheter kink or "pinching"
5. Other mechanical etiology
6. ? Venous thrombosis

Partial occlusion

↓

Port: Verify Huber needle placement by contact with needle stop

External: Connect syringe directly to hub

↓

Attempt to irrigate with 10 cc normal saline

↙ ↓ ↘

- Patient complains of pain (? catheter fracture)
- Resistance met
- Flushes without resistance or pain

Resistance met → Re-check needle placement → Resistance persists

Flushes without resistance or pain → Hang maintenance I.V. solution

Hang maintenance I.V. solution →
- Infusion varies
- Infuses normally and without variation depending on patient position → Proceed with treatment

Chest X-ray
Catheter contrast study
Possible venogram

If normal attempt to clear catheter (see Chapter 6)

APPENDIX E
Paradigm for the Evaluation and Treatment of Complete Catheter Occlusion

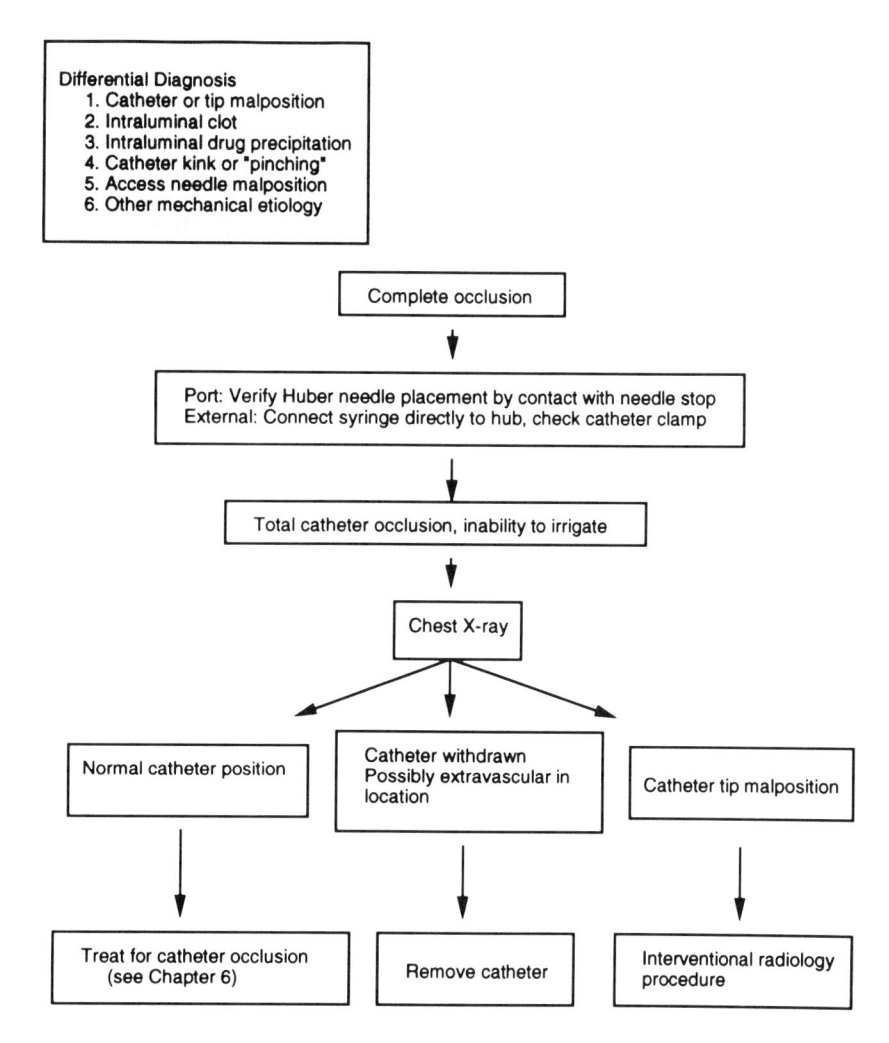

Differential Diagnosis
1. Catheter or tip malposition
2. Intraluminal clot
3. Intraluminal drug precipitation
4. Catheter kink or "pinching"
5. Access needle malposition
6. Other mechanical etiology

Complete occlusion
↓
Port: Verify Huber needle placement by contact with needle stop
External: Connect syringe directly to hub, check catheter clamp
↓
Total catheter occlusion, inability to irrigate
↓
Chest X-ray
↓

- Normal catheter position → Treat for catheter occlusion (see Chapter 6)
- Catheter withdrawn, Possibly extravascular in location → Remove catheter
- Catheter tip malposition → Interventional radiology procedure

APPENDIX F
Types and Initial Management of Catheter-Related Infections

Type of Infection	Presentation and Management
Exit Site	• Localized erythema + tenderness at the exit site; minimal purulence around catheter; systemic signs possible but not typical • Culture, local wound care, oral or i.v. antibiotics • If secondary to cuff extrusion catheter removal is necessary
Tunnel Infection	• Erythema, induration, and tenderness along the subcutaneous catheter track; purulence frequently seen at exit site; systemic signs frequent • Catheter must be removed; culture; i.v. antibiotics usually indicated • Tissue necrosis and worsening cellulitis can occur if not treated promptly
Pocket Infection	• Comparable to "tunnel infection" • Suppurative process around port housing; skin signs may be subtle • Diagnosis can be confirmed by aspirating fluid from around port housing • Port must be removed; pocket packed open, i.v. antibiotics usually indicated
Line-Sepsis	• Bacteremic sepsis secondary to infected intravascular portion of catheter • No evidence of another source for infection • Frequently a recent history of catheter manipulation • Obtain catheter and peripheral blood cultures; start i.v. antibiotics; if patient clinically stable the catheter can remain in-situ • For diagnostic criteria see Chapter 7

Index

The letter *f* following a page number indicates a figure; the letter *t* following a page number indicates a table.

A

Adenocarcinoma, lung, thrombosis rate associated with, 97–100
Adult patients, performance of ports versus external catheters, 32
Age
  and catheter dislodgement, pediatric patients, 49t
  and risk of infection, in pediatric patients, 30, 31t
Angiographic/surgical technique, 83–86, 83f, 84f, 85f
Antibiotic therapy
  in catheter-related sepsis, outcome, 120t
  flushing devices with vancomycin, 152–153
Azygos vein catheterization, 71–72, 72f, 73f

B

Bacteremia, catheter-related, 118–119
  treatment for, 119–122
Biofilm on long-term venous access catheters, 115
Bone marrow transplantation
  as an indication for external catheters, 34
  venous access catheters for patients, 39
Breakaway needle, 140–141f
Broviac catheters, 3
  failure-free interval, comparison with ports and Hickman catheters, 27
  performance of, selected reports, 24t
  placement of, retropleural approach to the azygos vein, 73f

C

Candida infections in pediatric patients with long-term venous access devices, 121
Candidemia, outcomes of treatment of amphotericin B, and catheter removal, 121t
Catheter occlusion, 77, 91–93, 159–160
Catheter-related infections
  with peripherally inserted central catheters, 144t
  types of, 113–114
  See also Complications
Catheter tip
  cultures of, direct Gram staining, 115
  location of
    azygos vein catheterization, 71–72, 72f, 73f
    and complications, 44
    saphenous vein catheterization, 76–77
Catheter tracking devices versus fluoroscopy, 136
Central venous catheters (CVCs), 3
  percutaneous, 12–14

Chemotherapy
    external catheters versus implantable ports for, 34
    single-lumen versus double-lumen catheters for, 20
    venous access catheters for, 39
Children's Cancer Study Group (CCSG), 31
Complications
    of direct venous access, femoral vein, 77
    of long-term venous access, 91–125
        prevention techniques, 157–158
        management of, 158–160
    of peripherally inserted central catheters, 142–144
    of peripherally inserted implantable ports, 145, 145t
    time to removal, pediatric patients, catheters and implantable ports, 28
Computed tomography (CT), diagnosis of catheter-related venous thrombosis, 101
Contraindications to central venous system access, 77
Costs
    of CVCs versus long-term venous catheters, 13–14
    of long-term venous access versus peripherally inserted central catheters, 144
    of removal, external catheter versus implanted port, 21
    total
        external catheter versus implanted port, 22
        of peripherally inserted central catheters, 142

D

Diagnosis
    of catheter-related infection, 116–119
    of catheter-related venous thrombosis, 100–101, 101t
Doppler sonography to diagnose thoracic inlet venous thrombosis, 100–101
Dormia basket catheter, 83
Double-lumen catheter, Hickman, 5–6
    for chemotherapy, 20
Double-lumen implantable ports, 10–11

E

Edema
    chronic extremity edema, in patients with venous thromboses, 96
    lower extremity, with inferior vena cava catheters, 77
Ethanol, for clearing lipid-containing occlusions, 92
Etiology
    of catheter-related bacteremia, 114–116
    of catheter-related venous thrombosis, 97–100
Exit site
    dressings for, 155t
    infections of, 113
        peripherally inserted central catheters, 144t
    maintenance of, 153–155
External catheters
    complications requiring removal, 26t
    versus implantable ports, 20–22
    indications for, 19–20
    maintenance of, 151–153
    performance of, selected reports, 24t
Extravasation, management of, 158–159

F

Femoral vein, catheterization via, 77, 78f
Fibrous ingrowth to hold catheters in place, 5
Fluoroscopy, to verify catheter placement, 41, 42, 47–48, 66, 76, 79
Fracture, of external catheters, 19

G

Gonadal vein, for access to the inferior vena cava, 80–81, 80f

Groshong catheter, 3, 6–8, 153
  repair of, 14
Guidewire insertion technique, 46

H

Hematological malignancies, indication for external catheters, 34
Hemostasis in internal jugular vein cutdown, 63, 66
Heparin, to reduce incidence of catheter-related venous thrombosis, 106
Hickman and Broviac catheters, 4–8
Hickman catheters, 3, 85f
  complications with
    infectious, 23–25
    noninfectious, 92t
    versus CVCs, random trial, 3
  double-lumen, 5–6
  failure-free interval, comparison with ports and Broviac catheters, 27
  insertion of
    angiographic/surgical technique, 83–84
    via the azygos vein, 71–72
  repair of, 14–15
  triple-lumen, 6
Home-based therapy
  home-based, 71
  peripherally inserted central catheters and, 142, 144
Huber needle, 13f
  for accessing implantable ports, 12, 21–22, 156–157
  placement of, 159f
Hydrochloric acid for clearing an occluded catheter, 90, 160

I

Implantable ports, 8–12
  accessing, 12, 21–23, 156–157
  complications with, 22, 22t
    requiring removal of, 26t
  double-lumen, 10–11
  versus external catheters, 20–22
  failure-free interval, comparison with Hickman and Breviac catheters, 27
  indications for, 19
  insertion of, 49
  occluded, urokinase therapy for, 94
  occlusion rate, prospective study, 10
  performance of, selected reports, 24
  removal of, 51–55
  risk of drug extravasation, 149–150
Incidence of catheter-related venous thrombosis, 97–100
Indications, for direct right atrial catheterization, 73–74
Infectious complications
  central venous catheters, 13
  double-lumen catheters, 20
  Hickman single-lumen and double-lumen catheters, 20t
  with long-term venous access devices, 113–125
  rate of
    Hickman versus CVCs, 4t
    implantable ports versus external catheters, 23, 27
    implantable ports versus Hickman/Broviac catheters, 25
    nontunneled long-term subclavian CVCs, 14t
  time to first infection, pediatric patients, 29f
Inferior epigastric vein, access to the inferior vena cava via, 77–79, 78f
Inferior vena cava
  access via the inferior epigastric vein, 77–79
  access via the lumbar vein, 81–82
  direct cannulation of, 82–83, 82f
  inguinal access, in pediatric patients, 75–79
Inguinal approaches to the inferior vena cava, 75–79
Insertion kit, venous access catheter, 9f
Insertion technique
  peripherally inserted central catheters, 136–141
  venous access catheters, 39–55
Intraluminal precipitation from drug mixtures, 92

Irrigation of an implantable port, 157

J

Jugular vein
  external cutdown, 50–51, 52f
  internal cutdown, 59–66

L

Leonard catheter, 3, 5–6
Line sepsis, 114
Longevity, external catheters and implantable ports, adult patients, 33
Lumbar vein, access to the inferior vena cava via, 81–82, 81f
Lumen occlusion, incidence of, adult patients, 32

M

Magnetic resonance imaging (MRI), sensitivity of, in catheter-related venous thrombosis diagnosis, 99
Maintenance program
  for central venous catheters, 13
  cost of, Groshong catheter, 6–8
  for implantable ports, 19
  and infectious complications, 3, 33, 34
  long-term venous access devices, 149–161
Mechanical failure in Hickman catheters, single-lumen and double-lumen, 21t
Memorial Sloan-Kettering Cancer Center
  clinical performance of Hickman catheters, with silver-impregnated cuff, 158
  clinical performance of Hickman catheters versus implanted ports, 32
  prospective evaluation, frequency of catheter evaluation, 152
Meta-analysis of transparent dressing, intravenous catheter sites, 153–154

Morbidity in thoracotomy-based techniques, 74–75
Mycobacteria, infection of tunnel or pocket by, 114
Mycobacterium fortuitum, catheter-related infection by, 122

N

Needle, breakaway, 140–141f
New technologies, 131–145

O

Occlusion
  of catheters, 89–91, 159–160
  withdrawal, 93
  with inferior vena cava catheters, 76
Occlusion rate, implantable ports, 10, 12

P

Parenteral infusion therapy
  home-based, 71
  long-term central venous access for, 86–87
Patient acceptance of implanted ports, 21
  pediatric patients, 27
Patient education, 160–161
  and inadvertent catheter removal, 23
  and infectious complications, 3, 34, 124
Patient selection for venous access catheters, 39–40
Pediatric patients
  catheter-related bacteremia, 119–120
  with long-term venous access devices, 118–119
  evaluation of antibiotic catheter flush, 124, 153
  implantable ports versus external catheters for, 26–32
  infectious complications, 115–116
  inguinal access to the inferior vena cava in, 77

peripherally inserted central catheters for, 132
urokinase therapy, for catheter-related venous thrombosis, 95, 103
Peel-away sheath, 139, 139f
Performance
of implantable ports versus catheters, adult patients, 32
of long-term venous access catheters, 19–34
of peripherally inserted central catheters, 142–144
of peripherally inserted implantable ports, 144–145
Peripherally inserted central catheters (PICCs), 131–145
efficacy and complications, selected reviews of, 143t
guidelines for estimating lengths, 138t
Peripherally inserted implanted port, 134–135
Persistent withdrawal occlusion (PWO), in implanted ports, 94
Plastic for implantable ports, 8–12
Platelet counts and thrombus formation, 100
Platelet transfusion, preparation for venous access catheter insertion, 40
Polyurethane central venous catheters, 13
peripherally inserted, 131
Pooled data, infectious complications with vascular access catheters, 33
Pott's occluding tie, 63
Preparation
for internal jugular vein cutdown, 59
for venous access catheter insertion, 39–40
Prophylaxis
to reduce catheter-related infections, 122–125, 158
to reduce catheter-related venous thrombosis, 105–107
Prospective studies
analysis of factors affecting infection rates, 27–28, 28t
rates of removal of external catheters and ports, pediatric patients, 31–32, 32t
See also Random trial
Pseudocapsule, over implantable port housing, 53–54f
Pulmonary embolism in patients with venous thromboses, 96

R

Radiology, interventional, to correct malposition of catheters, 93
Random trial
Hickman catheters
versus CVCs, 3
versus implantable ports, 23
of prophylactic antibiotics during catheter insertion, 124–125
of warfarin, for catheter-related venous thrombosis prevention, 106
Removal
indications for, external catheters or ports, 30t
reasons for, catheters versus ports, 33t
Repair kit, 14–15, 160
Resistance to flow for evaluation of an occluded catheter, 92
Retroperitoneal approach for access to the inferior central venous system, 79–83
Retrospective study, performance, Hickman/Broviac catheters versus implanted ports, 25
Right atrial catheterization, 73–74, 75f
Risks
of catheter-related venous thrombosis, 99
of infectious complications, central venous catheters, 13
of thrombosis, and tumor histology, 97–98, 98t

S

Saphenous vein, access to inferior vena cava, 76–77, 76f

Secondary thrombophlebitis in patients with venous thromboses, 96
Seldinger method, venous access catheter insertion, 41–42, 77
Sepsis with inferior vena cava catheters, 76
Septicemia, line-related
    Hickman catheters versus implantable ports, 25
    and neutrophil count, 40
    treatment of, 120
Sheath/dilator insertion, 46–47
Silastic
    for central venous catheters, 13–14, 32
    for glue, catheter repair, 15, 160
    for peripherally inserted central catheters, 131
    for thin-walled catheters, 8
Silicone
    alternative to polyvinyl chloride, 3
    in central venous catheters, 13, 94–95
    for diaphragm, for implantable ports, 8
Silver ion impregnated catheter cuff, evaluation of, 122–123, 158
Single-lumen catheters for chemotherapy, 20
Site selection
    peripherally inserted central catheters, 151
    venous access catheters, long-term, 40, 40t, 45–46
Squamous carcinoma, lung, thrombosis rate associated with, 97
Staphylococci, coagulase-negative, infections with, pediatric patients, 116
Staphylococcus aureus
    catheter-related infections, prognosis, 121–122
    cultured form hub and catheter tip samples, 117
    exit site infection by, 113
    pediatric patients, 116
Staphylococcus epidermis
    cultured form hub and catheter tip samples, 117
    exit site infection by, 113
Streptodornase for therapy, occluded venous access devices, 95

Streptokinase
    for catheter-related thromboses, 102–107
    management of occluded venous access devices, 95
Subclavian vein thrombosis, 97–100
    diagnosis of, 100–101
Subcutaneous ports, size of catheter, 3
Superior central venous system, 69f
Superior vena cava, catheterization of, 72–75, 74f
Surecath needle, 156

T

Technique
    internal jugular cutdown, 59–66
    percutaneous insertion, venous access catheters, 40–44
Teicoplanin, random trial of, for prophylaxis during catheter insertion, 125
Thoracic venous thrombosis, 99
Thoracotomy with direct catheterization, superior central venous system, 71
Thrombolytic therapy, 93–94, 94t
Thrombotic complications, external catheters versus implanted ports, 25
Timing of venous access catheter insertion, 39–40
Tissue plasminogen activator (t-PA) for treatment of occluded central venous catheters, 96, 96t
Titanium for implantable ports, 8–9
Treatment
    of catheter occlusion, 93–96
    of catheter-related venous thrombosis, 102–107
    of line sepsis, 119–122
Triple-lumen catheter, Hickman, 6
Tumor type, and risk of infection, in pediatric patients, 31t
Tunnel
    infections of, 113–114
    site and length, for venous access catheters, 48

U

Urokinase
  local therapy for catheter-related venous thrombosis, 102–103
  responses to, catheter-related venous thrombosis, 105t
  therapy for occluded venous access devices, 94–95, 94t

V

Vancomycin with heparin, to flush catheters, 124, 152–153
Venography to establish patency of the inferior vena cava, 80
Venous access catheter insertion, 39–55
  kit for, 9f
Venous patency, establishing, before central venous catheter insertion, 71–72

Venous thrombosis
  in adult patients, 32
  catheter occlusion with, 93
  catheter-related, 96–107
  correlation with catheter tip placement, 26, 26t
  with double lumen catheters, 20
  in Hickman catheters, single-lumen and double-lumen, 21t

W

Warfarin, for catheter-related venous thrombosis prevention, 106–107
Withdrawal occlusion, 93, 159
  incidence of, adult patients, 32

X

X-ray, to identify cause of catheter occlusion, 92

ISBN 0-397-51316-X